# NATURAL THERAPIES

## *for*

# EMPHYSEMA

## *and*

# COPD

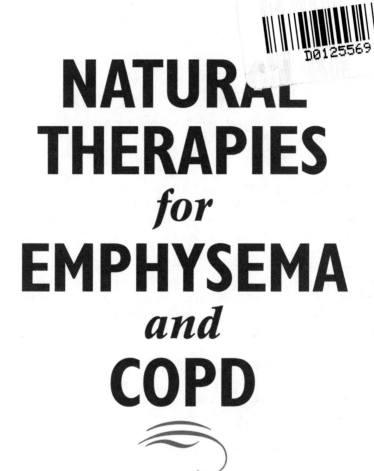

*Relief and Healing for*
*Chronic Pulmonary Disorders*

## ROBERT J. GREEN JR., ND

Healing Arts Press
Rochester, Vermont

Healing Arts Press
One Park Street
Rochester, Vermont 05767
www.HealingArtsPress.com

Healing Arts Press is a division of Inner Traditions International

*Note to the reader: This book is intended as an informational guide. The remedies,
approaches, and techniques described herein are meant to supplement, and not to
be a substitute for, professional medical care or treatment. They should not be used
to treat a serious ailment without prior consultation with a qualified health care
professional.*

**Library of Congress Cataloging-in-Publication Data**

Green, Robert J., Jr.
  Natural therapies for emphysema and COPD : relief and healing for chronic
pulmonary disorders / Robert J. Green Jr.
      p. cm.
  Includes bibliographical references and index.
  ISBN-13: 978-1-59477-163-7
  ISBN-10: 1-59477-163-4
  1. Emphysema, Pulmonary—Alternative treatment. 2. Lungs—Diseases,
Obstructive—Alternative treatment. 3. Self-care, Health. I. Title.
  RC776.E5.G74 2007
  616.2'48—dc22

                                                                2007004116

Printed and bound in Canada by Transcontinental Printing

10  9  8  7  6  5  4  3  2  1

Text design by Rachel Goldenberg and layout by Priscilla Baker
This book was typeset in Sabon, with Galaxie used as a display typeface
Illustrations by Dan Woodward

To send correspondence to the author of this book, mail a first-class letter to the
author c/o Inner Traditions • Bear & Company, One Park Street, Rochester, VT
05767, and we will forward the communication.

*To my father, Robert Green Sr., whose personal
battle with laryngeal cancer and COPD inspired me
to write this book.*

*To my wife, Patricia, whose virtue no words can
describe, and my children, John, Zarah, and Joseph.
You are my joy.*

*To Mr. and Mrs. Francesco Caccavale, without
whose support this book could not have
been written.*

*And to the Lord, in whom all healing is found.
You are my light and my truth.*

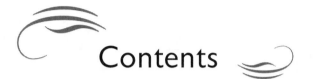

# Contents

# Acknowledgments

I offer my sincerest thanks to all of my former professors and to every person who was instrumental in bringing this manuscript to fruition. The following individuals are deserving of special mention, as their contributions to my life have been invaluable. Collectively, they taught me how to think critically and how to appropriately apply reason in formulating meaningful questions. Their tireless dedication to teaching and academic excellence will forever remain the bar against which I measure myself. But perhaps most important—through the impact of their kindness and selfless humility, I became a better person by knowing them. For all they have given me, I am forever grateful.

Robert F. Good, MD
*(In memoriam)*

John Kotselas, MA
*Author and Lecturer in Theology*

William Cheek, PhD
*Professor Emeritus of History*

Herbert Lebherz, PhD
*Professor Emeritus of Biochemistry*

Robert Waters, PhD
*Professor of Biochemistry*

Sharon Satterfield, ND
*Doctor of Naturopathy*

Henry Shatz, MA
*Professor of Spanish*

# Introduction

Chronic obstructive pulmonary disease, commonly called COPD, describes a group of debilitating diseases that cause serious problems with breathing. An estimated 35 million people in the United States have one form or another of COPD, a category that includes emphysema, chronic bronchitis, and other serious respiratory problems. COPD is the fourth leading cause of death in America, claiming nearly 120,000 lives annually. In 2004, COPD care cost the United States more than $37 billion. The number of people with COPD worldwide is as high as 293 million.

Most cases of emphysema and chronic bronchitis are related to cigarette smoking, but a genetic disorder and inhalation of toxic substances can also play a role. Those who either live with COPD or take care of someone with serious respiratory problems know all too well the high price these people pay in their daily efforts to survive and carry on with life. Despite the best of intentions, conventional medicine is still quite limited in what it can offer to help with COPD. Conventional treatment for COPD most often consists of the use of powerful drugs to control inflammation and keep the airways open. These drugs can cause serious side effects and do not slow the progression of the disease.

There are alternatives to the use of strong pharmaceutical drugs to treat COPD, and that is the subject of this book. Natural medicine—nutritional change, dietary supplements, herbs, and physical therapies—can ease symptoms of COPD and improve the underlying problems that cause the symptoms. Perhaps best of all, by improving the health of your whole body—not just your lungs—the simple methods I describe in this book will enhance your well-being and quality of life for years to come.

My interest and subsequent passion to help people with COPD began more than a decade ago, when my father started to manifest the symptoms of COPD, a condition that had been diagnosed much earlier in his life. As I took care of him and became more involved in researching alternatives to conventional medical treatment, the career path in medicine that I had envisioned took on a new face. I realized that focusing on natural medicine—including nutrition, dietary supplements, and the wisdom of traditional medical systems around the world—would allow me to make the greatest contribution to helping people improve their health and quality of life. I became convinced that the true key to addressing chronic disease lies in embracing the principles of natural medicine and applying natural approaches to health and living.

There is no question that modern medicine has given us many life-saving technologies and drugs. Pharmaceutical drugs are sometimes necessary to get symptoms under control. However, it was the integration of nutritional and natural therapeutics into my father's treatment plan that made the most significant difference in his health. My father did not begin utilizing natural medicine to care for his COPD until the age of sixty-nine, but it is clear to all involved in his health care, including his conventional physicians, that it was the implementation of natural health methods that enabled him to survive and have a much improved quality of life until he went to his final rest at the age of eighty-three.

My years of study and research have drawn upon both conventional and natural medical methods and philosophies. I have thoroughly enjoyed the puzzle-solving and scientific detective work inherent in research, and it has deepened my appreciation for the scientific basis of natural medicine. Reflecting on the research and study I have done, I realized that by writing about natural approaches to health, I could reach infinitely more people with the useful information they need to improve their health than I ever could through my private practice alone. This is why I have decided to make writing about the natural approaches to health an integral part of my career.

I subscribe to the idea that the knowledge and practice of nutrition and natural health care should be accessible not only to professional health care practitioners, but also to the general public. While some of the material in this book is technical, I have done my best to explain it in terms anyone can understand. I've included a glossary of unfamiliar terms, and suggestions for further reading in appendix 2.

Natural medicine is not a panacea or miracle cure for COPD, and this book is by no means an exhaustive source of all that is known about the respiratory system, COPD, or natural treatments for COPD. It is my hope, however, that the information I've assembled here will help you understand the processes behind the development of COPD and how natural therapeutics may be used to change the course of the disease.

## THE PRINCIPLES OF NATURAL HEALTH CARE

Natural health is a way of life, not just a way of healing illness. It involves living according to a set of principles that require us to seek balance in our lives and recognize our responsibility for our own health. The modern American lifestyle is usually at odds with these principles, but if you learn to slow down and pay attention to your body, you will have taken the first step on the road to better health.

Natural health care is often referred to as "holistic" health care. The word *holistic,* derived from *whole,* refers to systems of health care that take into account the needs of the whole person, not just the symptoms of a disease. Thus, holistic health care aims to build the health and well-being of the whole person and is tailored to meet each individual's needs with diet and lifestyle changes as well as specific treatments.

My particular focus in natural health care is traditional naturopathy, a branch of holistic health care that emphasizes dietary modification, nutritional supplementation, herbs, bodywork and other physical therapies, and attention to emotional and spiritual issues as well as physical problems. Traditional naturopaths are primarily teachers who educate clients on approaches to healthful living and building health through noninvasive natural means. Naturopathy itself is a philosophy of life and an approach to living. The philosophy suggests we should live a lifestyle as close to nature as possible, which includes consuming food from natural sources, drinking pure water, breathing fresh air, enjoying the warmth of sunshine, exercising the body regularly in natural ways, and obtaining adequate rest.

At the heart of all holistic health systems is a focus on building health, not just treating or managing disease. Proponents of natural health practices have always understood that when you eliminate toxins and give the body what it needs to function properly, disease and other physical problems typically resolve themselves. In 1997, Americans spent $27 billion on alternative medicine, the majority of which was spent out of pocket. Surely this is testimony to the fact that Americans are ready for alternatives to conventional health care and its focus on treating disease rather than building wellness.

## HOW TO USE THIS BOOK

I wrote this book to offer guidance to people who are sincerely seeking answers and help with COPD from the arena of natural and alternative medicine. The dietary changes and natural remedies introduced here are designed to be used in concert with one another. Dietary change is the foundation upon which all other therapeutic methods are built.

This book is not intended as a self-help guide. COPD is serious and requires diagnosis and care from a qualified health care practitioner. I wrote this book primarily for people who have already been diagnosed with COPD and their loved ones, as well as anyone else interested in learning about how to use natural health principles to improve symptoms of COPD and rebuild health. If you have been diagnosed with COPD, I urge you to find a qualified natural health practitioner who can help you implement the guidelines set forth here. Any doctor educated in holistic health philosophies and treatment methods should be most willing to work with you to implement the techniques and strategies outlined in this book. If your current doctor is unwilling to work with you in incorporating the dietary changes, supplements, and physical therapies I recommend, see appendix 1 for a list of organizations that can help you find a qualified health care practitioner in your area.

Nutrition is the cornerstone of natural healing for COPD. The degree of success you achieve with all other natural therapeutic methods will be directly proportional to your ability to adhere to the dietary changes I recommend. As you begin to become comfortable with your new eating habits and see the progress you are making in improving your condition, you can begin to add herbs and other dietary supplements to your health-building program. Exercise and other physical therapies round out this basic approach to building health. By giving your body these essentials, you will not only improve your symptoms, you will also be giving your body all of the elements it needs to heal itself. This is one of the central premises of naturopathy—assisting the body in its quest to heal itself.

By creating an optimal internal environment through nutrition, herbs, supplements, and exercise, you allow other forms of natural medicine such as homeopathy and acupuncture to be of maximum benefit to you. Natural health care offers myriad ways to address the health issues faced by people with COPD, from breathlessness and excess mucus production to frequent infections and lack of energy.

The following list outlines the therapeutic goals most COPD patients would like to be able to accomplish. The nutritional methods available to address these issues are abundant. As you begin to make changes in the way you eat, and begin to introduce nutritional supplements, herbs, and gentle exercise into your lifestyle, keep these goals in mind so you can monitor your progress in the areas that matter most to you.

Therapeutic goals (not necessarily in order of priority):

- Repair and heal damaged tissue to whatever extent possible
- Increase breathing capacity, with greater airflow through the airways
- Manage and control mucus production
- Manage and control inflammation
- Prevent infection and strengthen immunity

- Increase vitality
- Increase ability to exercise and exert energy
- Decrease dependency on pharmaceutical drugs as much as possible
- Improve overall health status

Natural health methods can help you achieve all of these goals, but you must be patient and allow your body the time it needs to rebuild itself. Healing takes time, so don't expect to see instantaneous results. Much will depend upon the status of your health at the time you begin implementing natural health practices and how faithfully you follow natural health guidelines. Some of you will start to see improvement after a few weeks or a month, and others will not start seeing any improvement until later. Plan to allow yourself at least one to three months of following my guidelines before expecting to see any significant improvement in your condition.

Based on my experience and research, I am confident that if you follow the strategies outlined in this book, and work with a qualified health care provider who can provide skillful guidance, you will be able to breathe more easily, your overall health will improve, and you will be well on your way to a better quality of life within just a few months. May you be blessed and encouraged as you begin the process of building your health.

# 1

# Essential Respiratory Anatomy and Physiology

The respiratory system is a marvelously complex system that maintains one of the most vital functions of the human body: breathing. The well-being of the entire body is vitally dependent upon proper functioning of every detail of respiration—the process by which the body takes in oxygen, distributes oxygen to cells throughout the body, and releases carbon dioxide created as a by-product of the process. The respiratory system must not only operate efficiently, it must also protect itself from environmental irritants and infection. The main purpose of the lungs is to facilitate the exchange of oxygen from the air we breathe with carbon dioxide given off by the cells of the body. The blood circulation transports oxygen to the cells of the body and carries carbon dioxide back to the lungs to be exhaled in the breath. Thus, the heart and circulatory system also play a vital role in respiration.

Respiration is a four-phase process. The first phase of respiration is breathing, otherwise known as pulmonary ventilation. Breathing consists of inspiration (inhaling) and expiration (exhaling) of air. This vital function is controlled by brain structures called the medulla oblongata and the pons. These structures, which are located in the brain stem portion of the central nervous system, send nerve impulses that stimulate the muscles that control the breathing process (the thoracic muscles and the diaphragm). The nervous system control of breathing is predominantly an involuntary (automatic) process, but can be voluntarily controlled as needed. The voluntary aspect is best evidenced in the interruption of breathing when you cough or when you hold your breath, for example.

In the second phase of respiration, technically known as pulmonary or external respiration, an exchange of oxygen and carbon dioxide gases occurs between the lungs and the blood. Oxygen is transferred from the lungs into the blood to be distributed to tissues all over the body. At the same time, carbon dioxide is removed from the blood to be exhaled in the breath. Efficient oxygen transfer depends on the presence of sufficient amounts of hemoglobin in the red blood cells, which are responsible for carrying oxygen from the lungs to the tissues. This is why individuals who are anemic, having lower than optimal amounts of hemoglobin, have additional concerns that complicate their COPD issues.

The third phase of respiration, which does not take place in the lungs, is called internal (tissue) respiration. This phase involves the exchange of gases between the blood and the tissues of the body.

The fourth and final phase of respiration, cellular respiration, occurs inside the body's cells. Through the process of cellular respiration, the body uses the oxygen that has been obtained from the blood to make energy and sustain metabolic activity. As part of this process, the body generates carbon dioxide as a waste product.

## GENERAL ANATOMY OF THE LUNGS

The lungs are elastic, spongelike organs that lie in the thoracic cavity (the chest). The lungs are enclosed within the rib cage. The top of the lungs reaches slightly above the clavicle (collarbone), and the base of the lungs, which is slightly curved, fits over the diaphragm (a muscular structure that separates the chest cavity from the abdominal cavity). The right lung is somewhat shorter than the left to accommodate the space needed by the liver, which lies just below the diaphragm under the right lung.

A two-layered membrane composed mainly of elastic tissue (the pleural membrane) encloses and protects the lungs within the thoracic cavity. The inner membrane, called the visceral pleura, lines the lungs

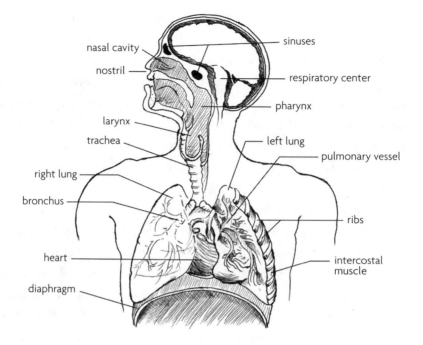

*Fig. 1. The respiratory system and related structures.*

themselves. The outer membrane, the parietal pleura, is attached to the wall of the thoracic cavity. A thin film of fluid (called pleural fluid) occupies the space between the two membranes in order that their surfaces can easily slide over one another during inspiration and expiration.

The right lung consists of three lobes and the left lung has two. The right lung is also divided into ten sections and the left into nine sections. These sectional subdivisions amount to what can be thought of as a three-dimensional map that allows for greater precision in specifying locations within the lungs.

## PATHWAY OF AIRFLOW THROUGH THE RESPIRATORY SYSTEM

The respiratory system begins at the nostrils, where air enters the nasal cavity and proceeds into the nasopharynx (the passage that connects the nose with the throat). As air passes through the structures of the nasal cavity, it is filtered by coarse nasal hairs and warmed and humidified by a highly vascularized mucous membrane. From the nasopharynx, the air continues down the oropharynx and the laryngopharynx (the back of the mouth and the throat) through the larynx (voice box) into the trachea (windpipe). The trachea is a tube constructed of cartilage that extends down from the larynx about four inches. At this point, it divides into two branches, called the primary bronchial tubes. These—the right and left primary bronchi—are the first two main branches of the bronchial tree.

Where the primary bronchi enter the lungs, they begin branching into smaller bronchi called secondary or lobar bronchi. These secondary bronchi divide and branch into tertiary bronchi, which further divide into even smaller tubes called bronchioles, which themselves continue to divide into smaller branches. Bronchioles eventually become tiny terminal bronchioles that give rise to branches of respiratory bronchioles. These respiratory bronchioles ultimately end in clusters of air sacs that contain individual alveoli.

Alveoli are tiny air-containing cavities at the endpoint of the respiratory passageways in the lungs. Each lung has roughly 300 million alveoli

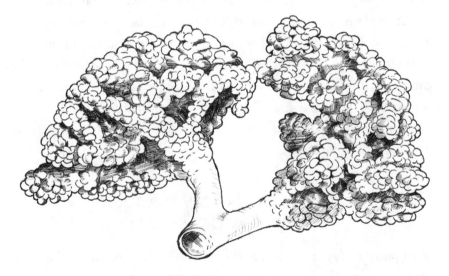

*Fig. 2. Two acini, showing a terminal bronchiole splitting into two respiratory bronchioles with alveolar ducts and alveoli.*

and each one of them is essentially a gas bubble that is surrounded by a network of capillaries (tiny blood vessels).

Alveoli are connected to the respiratory bronchioles by passageways called alveolar ducts. Two or more alveoli that share a common alveolar duct are called alveolar sacs.

Terminal bronchioles along with their respective respiratory bronchioles and alveolar sacs are known as lobules. Respiratory bronchioles and their alveolar sacs are collectively known as the acinus. The acinus is essentially a lobule without the terminal bronchiole, and it is where actual gas exchange in the lungs occurs. The acinus is something like a cluster of grapes, in which the main stem coming off the vine is the respiratory bronchiole, the smaller stems are the alveolar ducts, and the grapes themselves represent the alveoli.

### TABLE 1. STRUCTURES OF THE PATHWAY OF AIRFLOW THROUGH THE RESPIRATORY SYSTEM

1. Nasal cavity
2. Pharynx (nasopharynx, oropharynx, laryngopharynx)
3. Larynx
4. Trachea
5. Left and right primary bronchi
6. Secondary (lobar) bronchi
7. Tertiary bronchi
8. Bronchioles
9. Terminal bronchioles
10. Respiratory bronchioles
11. Alveolar ducts
12. Alveolar sacs
13. Individual alveoli

Structures 9 through 13 constitute a lobule. Structures 10 through 13 constitute an acinus (the site of gas exchange).

The alveoli are separated from one another by membranes called the interalveolar septa (a matrix consisting of connective tissue fibers and capillaries), and are connected to each other by what are known as pores of Kohn. These pores are essentially holes that exist between the alveoli that allow for the complete ventilation of air throughout the acinus. It is essential to realize that there is no truly free space between the alveoli. They are always surrounded by a matrix of connective tissue fibers and capillaries—the interalveolar septum.

## STRUCTURAL SUPPORT OF THE RESPIRATORY SYSTEM

From the trachea to the bronchioles, the respiratory tract is supported primarily by rings and plates made of cartilage (tough, elastic tissue). The cartilage disappears in the bronchioles, as bronchioles themselves are not supported by cartilage, but rather are surrounded by smooth muscle, which allows for fluctuation in the size of the bronchiole. Bronchioles are also characterized by the presence of elastic fibers that surround them in addition to the smooth muscle.

## BLOOD SUPPLY TO THE LUNGS

There are two separate systems of blood flow in the lungs: pulmonary circulation and bronchial. The first of these two systems, pulmonary circulation, involves the blood that circulates from the heart through the pulmonary blood vessels. This is the part of the circulatory system that picks up oxygen from the lungs, transports it to the tissues throughout the body, and returns the blood back to the lungs after the oxygen has been depleted by the tissues. The returning blood contains carbon dioxide excreted by the tissues as a waste product of metabolism.

As oxygen-rich blood circulates from the lungs throughout the body, the tissues take the oxygen they need from the blood. Thus the blood that is returned to the heart is essentially without oxygen. The heart sends this deoxygenated blood to the lungs by way of the pulmonary artery, through which it reaches the capillaries that surround the alveoli. Here, at the interface between the alveoli and capillaries, the blood receives a fresh supply of oxygen. After passing through the alveolar capillaries, the freshly oxygenated blood makes its way back to the heart by way of the pulmonary vein, where it then exits the heart through the aorta (a major artery) and circulates through another cycle of delivering oxygen to the tissues of the body. Upon receiving this fresh supply of oxygen, the tissues are now able to take care of their metabolic business. Carbon dioxide is one of the waste products of metabolism and the tissues will deliver carbon dioxide back into the bloodstream, where it will be carried back to the lungs and exhaled out of the body.

You may have learned that arteries are blood vessels that carry oxygen-rich blood away from the heart to the rest of the body and veins are blood vessels that carry oxygen-poor blood from the tissues back to the heart. This is mostly correct. However, the definition of an artery or vein actually hinges on the direction of blood flow toward or away from the heart, not the oxygen content of the blood the vessel carries. The pulmonary artery, for example, carries deoxygenated blood away from the heart. The pulmonary vein, which transports oxygen-rich blood from the alveolar capillaries in the lungs, is still a vein because it is taking blood toward the heart.

The second system of blood flow in the lungs, bronchial circulation, involves the circulation of blood through the blood vessels that nourish the lung tissue itself. The bronchial arteries receive oxygenated blood mainly from the aorta, and deliver this oxygen-rich blood to the lung tissue (e.g., the bronchi and bronchioles and the bronchial lymph nodes) via the capillaries adjacent to the cells of these tissues. After the lung tissue takes the oxygen it needs from the bronchial arteries, some of the now deoxygenated blood is returned to the heart by way of the bronchial veins and some by way of the pulmonary veins.

# LINING OF THE RESPIRATORY TRACT
# AND THE ALVEOLI

The respiratory tract is lined by a membrane called the respiratory epithelium. Epithelium is one of the four primary tissue types of the body. Epithelium lines the skin as well as internal organs and hollow cavities such as the intestines and the respiratory passageways. Epithelial cells line the insides of the lungs. The nasal cavity, nasopharynx, and other parts of the respiratory system (from the larynx to the bronchioles, but not including the vocal cords) are lined by a membrane containing epithelial cells with many mucus-secreting goblet cells. There are also many other mucus-secreting glands throughout the walls of the trachea and the bronchi, but not the bronchioles. These cells and glands help "condition" inhaled air to keep the respiratory system clean and free of particles.

Moist mucus secreted by these cells and glands traps foreign matter. At the same time, cilia (tiny hairlike structures) on the epithelium sweep away particles so that they may be swallowed or expectorated. This is the natural course of action for maintaining the respiratory passageways. Water to humidify inhaled air is derived from mucus, and heat to warm the air comes from the abundant underlying blood vessels. These processes work together to ensure that the air that travels through the respiratory tract is not only at body temperature, but also as clean as possible, and completely humidified.

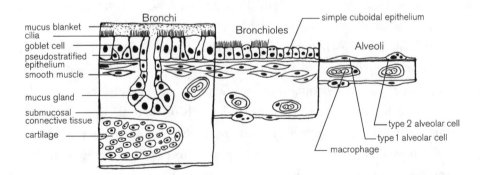

Fig. 3. The overall changes in the structure of the lining of the respiratory tract.

From the bronchioles onward, the branching network of the lungs becomes very extensive, and the nature of the cells lining the respiratory tract gradually begins to change. Once we reach the terminal bronchioles, the cells lining the respiratory tract no longer produce mucus, nor do they have cilia, and an immune system cell known as a macrophage assumes the responsibility of removing inhaled foreign particles. Rather than trapping and sweeping away foreign matter like cilia, macrophages engulf and digest the particles. As the terminal bronchioles eventually become respiratory bronchioles, the cells lining the respiratory tract change yet again into a cell type known as squamous epithelium, the same kind of cells that line the alveolar wall.

The walls of the alveoli are composed of only a single layer of cells, and they lie immediately next to capillaries that also consist of only a single layer of cells. The alveolar wall also contains its own macrophages, which are responsible for removing dust particles and other debris from the alveoli. Because the inner surface of the alveoli is moist and comes in direct contact with air (gas), the watery surface of the inner alveolar wall is always attempting to contract—much in the way water holds itself together on the rim of a glass that is about to overflow. This contracting force exhibited by the watery inner alveolar surface makes for a naturally existing surface tension at the liquid–gas interface of the inner alveolar wall. In effect, this tension inadvertently forces air out of the alveoli through the bronchioles, thus promoting the collapse of the alveoli. To compensate for this phenomenon, certain alveolar cells secrete a fluid that contains a surfactant that lowers the surface tension of the liquid–gas barrier and prevents the alveoli from collapsing upon exhalation.

## GAS EXCHANGE IN THE ALVEOLI

Successful exchange and efficient transport of oxygen and carbon dioxide are critical to sustaining the immediate cellular requirements of life. In one way or another, emphysema, chronic bronchitis, bronchiectasis, and the complications of infections and pneumonia all obstruct the airway and compromise the effectiveness of gas exchange. Many of the problems associated with emphysema occur in the part of the lungs in which gas exchange actually occurs (the acinus). As the airway obstructions that are characteristic of COPD interfere with gas exchange, the task of keeping the airway open with minimal obstruction is of primary importance.

The exchange of oxygen and carbon dioxide occurs across the alveolar and capillary walls. The actual movement of oxygen and carbon dioxide across these membranes is accomplished by a process called diffusion. Diffusion in this case means the movement of molecules from an area of higher concentration of that kind of molecule to an area of lower concentration. Simply put, this means a gas will move in the direction from where it is more concentrated to an area where it is less concentrated. Spraying air freshener into a room provides a classic example of this phenomenon. When the can is sprayed, the area immediately outside the can is densely concentrated with air freshener molecules, and this is where you can smell the fragrance most strongly. Over time, however, you will eventually be able to smell the fragrance on the other side of

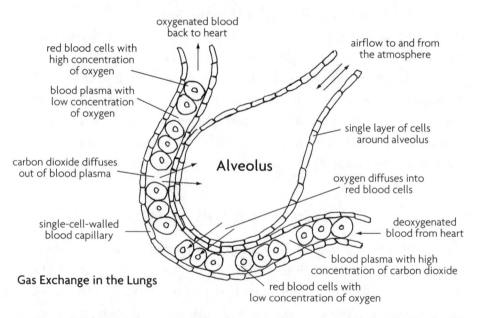

oxygenated blood
back to heart

red blood cells with
high concentration
of oxygen

blood plasma with
low concentration
of oxygen

airflow to and from
the atmosphere

single layer of cells
around alveolus

carbon dioxide diffuses
out of blood plasma

Alveolus

oxygen diffuses into
red blood cells

single-cell-walled
blood capillary

deoxygenated
blood from heart

blood plasma with high
concentration of carbon dioxide

Gas Exchange in the Lungs

red blood cells with
low concentration of oxygen

Fig. 4. Exchange of oxygen and carbon dioxide between the alveolus (hollow space) and the surrounding capillary.

the room. This is because the air freshener molecules diffused across the room to areas of lower concentration.

In the lungs, the concentration of oxygen and carbon dioxide is measured in terms of *partial pressures*. The partial pressure of a gas is simply a measure of its concentration in air or a liquid. Gases always expand to fill the container they are in, whether it is a room or a microscopic-sized alveolus. They also always diffuse from areas of higher concentration or pressure to areas of lower concentration or pressure. The partial pressure of oxygen in the lungs is much higher than the partial pressure of oxygen in the blood that is passing through the alveolar capillaries.

When blood returns to the lungs through the alveolar capillaries after it has circulated throughout the body, it contains very little oxygen. Because the concentration of oxygen in the blood in the alveolar capillaries is so low, a pressure gradient exists between the high oxygen concentration in the alveoli and the low oxygen concentration in the blood of the alveolar capillaries. Based on this pressure gradient, oxygen diffuses from the alveoli of the lungs (the area of higher concentration or partial pressure) into the blood (the area of lower concentration or partial pressure).

The exact reverse is true for carbon dioxide ($CO_2$). Carbon dioxide, the waste product of cellular metabolism, is continuously diffusing from the cells into the bloodstream. This means that the concentration of carbon dioxide in the alveolar capillaries is higher than in the lungs, and therefore the concentration or pressure gradient of carbon dioxide is in the opposite direction of oxygen. Because its concentration is higher in

### TABLE 2. RELATIONSHIP BETWEEN PARTIAL PRESSURE AND DIRECTION OF GAS FLOW

| Gas | Partial Pressure (mmHg) | | Direction of Gas Flow |
|---|---|---|---|
| | In lungs (alveoli) | In deoxygenated blood (alveolar capillaries—arterial side) | |
| Oxygen | 105 | 40 | From lungs into blood |
| Carbon dioxide | 40 | 45 | From blood into lungs |

the blood, carbon dioxide diffuses from the alveolar capillaries (area of higher concentration of carbon dioxide) into the alveoli of the lungs (area of lower concentration of carbon dioxide), where it is then exhaled.

Many sophisticated mechanisms tightly monitor and control every detail of gas exchange between the lungs and the blood. The vast majority (98 percent) of the oxygen that diffuses into the blood is transported by way of being bound to iron-rich hemoglobin on red blood cells. The binding of oxygen to hemoglobin and its subsequent transport to the tissues is itself a very complex process that is under strict regulation. Although some carbon dioxide is also transported by hemoglobin (about 23 percent), the majority of carbon dioxide is transported in the form of bicarbonate. Bicarbonate ($HCO_3^-$) is the substance formed when carbon dioxide reacts with water, and this too is a very tightly controlled process that maintains the proper blood concentrations of carbon dioxide.

$$CO_2 + H_2O \leftrightarrows H^+ + HCO_3^-$$

## THE MECHANICS OF BREATHING AND CONTROL OF RESPIRATION

Breathing (also known as pulmonary ventilation) is accomplished through the actions of several muscle groups. These muscle groups are stimulated by nerve impulses that emanate from the respiratory center deep in the brain, in the medulla and the pons. The main muscles involved with inspiration (inhaling) are the diaphragm, which is stimulated by the phrenic nerve, and the external intercostals (muscles between the ribs), which are stimulated by the intercostal nerves. Other muscles used in inspiration are the sternocleidomastoid and the scalenes, both of which are in the neck.

As explained previously, the nervous system control of breathing is predominantly an involuntary (automatic) process, but can be voluntarily controlled as needed. Overall regulation of breathing is controlled by neural and chemical reflex systems whose aim is to maintain the proper balance of oxygen delivery to, and carbon dioxide removal from, the tissues of the body.

The respiratory center in the brain stem is divided into three areas. The main area, called the medullary rhythmicity area, is located in the medulla oblongata. Neurons (nerves) in this part of the brain set the basic automatic rhythm of respiration. Neurons within this area spontaneously generate nerve impulses that initiate inspiration. These nerve impulses travel via the phrenic nerve to the diaphragm and via the intercostal nerves to the external intercostal muscles, causing contraction of these muscles, which results in inspiration. Contraction of the diaphragm and the external intercostal muscles increases the size of the thoracic cavity, and in so doing effectively creates a pressure differential whereby the pressure inside the chest cavity is now lower than the atmospheric pressure outside such that air flows into the lungs. Remember that gases flow in the direction of higher pressure to areas of lower pressure.

Nervous system regulation limits the time of the contraction of the diaphragm and the external intercostal muscles to just a couple of seconds, after which they relax until the next cycle. With the lungs now full of air, and the relaxation of the inspiratory muscles causing the size of the chest cavity to be reduced, you have a situation in which the pressure is higher inside the lungs—the opposite of before. As a result of the pressure differential being reversed, expiration occurs—in other words, air flows out of the lungs. Expiration during quiet breathing is normally passive, as there are no muscular contractions involved. Expiration is accomplished through the elastic recoil of the lungs and the chest wall. During labored breathing, other rib muscles and abdominal muscles become involved to forcibly expel air.

There are several other coordinating mechanisms that the body uses to either increase or decrease the rate of respiration. Changes in the pH of the blood, increased levels of carbon dioxide in the blood, elevated body temperature, or sudden severe pain will send messages to the respiratory center, where the respiratory rate is adjusted to meet the current needs of the body.

## *Nerve Supply to the Lungs*

Breathing is regulated by the autonomic nervous system (ANS), which controls involuntary body functions (such as the activity of heart muscle, smooth muscle, and glands). The nerves of the ANS are made up of both sympathetic and parasympathetic nerve fibers. Sympathetic fibers are usually associated with the "fight-or-flight" response. They generally have a stimulating effect on organs and body systems and are responsible for rapid sensory activity and movement. Parasympathetic fibers are usually associated with the "rest-and-digest" response and generally have a relaxing effect on the body. ANS parasympathetic motor nerve impulses produce smooth muscle bronchoconstriction (narrowing of the bronchi or bronchioles) and vasodilation (widening of the blood vessels) and promote secretion by the glands of the bronchial tree. ANS sympathetic motor nerve impulses cause smooth muscle bronchodilation (widening of the bronchi or bronchioles) and vasoconstriction (narrowing of the blood vessels) and inhibit gland secretion.

The respiratory system is a marvelously complex system that maintains one of the most vital functions of the human body. Some of the information in this chapter is quite technical, but it is not necessary to understand all of it in order to proceed with improving your health with natural medicine. Having an overall familiarity with the basic structure and function of the respiratory system may be useful in later chapters as you learn about the various forms of COPD. It also may enable you to understand more clearly the particulars of your individual case and how and why natural and alternative methods can be employed to help with your situation.

# 2

# Understanding COPD and Emphysema

Chronic obstructive pulmonary disease, commonly known as COPD, involves many complex and often overlapping problems in the respiratory system. The term COPD encompasses chronic bronchitis, emphysema, and other serious respiratory problems, including bronchiectasis (the irreversible dilation and distortion of the bronchi and bronchioles). Technically speaking, asthma is also in the COPD category, but COPD usually refers to emphysema or chronic bronchitis.

One factor all of these conditions have in common is that they are chronic, meaning that they developed slowly and have persisted over a long period of time. In addition, almost all cases of COPD affect people who smoked at least a pack of cigarettes a day for twenty years or more. Most exceptions to this general rule are rare cases involving people who have a genetic (inherited) condition called alpha-1 antitrypsin deficiency. However, individuals who have experienced long-term continual exposure to noxious substances can also manifest the symptoms of COPD. This is most often seen in people who have worked in chemical factories, coal mining, and other types of occupations where there is continous exposure to a substance that is an irritant to the respiratory system. The vast majority of COPD cases, however, are still a result of a history of cigarette smoking.

Chronic bronchitis and emphysema cause similar problems with breathing, and elements of both diseases usually are present to varying degrees in a person with COPD. In many cases, individuals have symptoms of both conditions because of the common underlying feature of cigarette smoking.

COPD takes a toll not only on the lungs, but also on many other essential organs and body systems, including the heart and circulatory system and the liver. Cor pulmonale (an abnormal enlargement of the right ventricle of the heart) commonly occurs with chronic bronchitis, and it is also seen in advanced emphysema. The liver, the body's main organ of detoxification, may become overwhelmed processing the toxins contained in cigarette smoke and pharmaceutical drugs.

The development of COPD is gradual. The disease typically begins during a person's forties, after a long history of cigarette smoking. Emphysema and chronic bronchitis share a number of signs and symptoms, including shortness of breath (dyspnea), chronic obstruction of the airflow through the lungs, and a reduced ability to expel air from the lungs. Emphysema affects the acinus (the part of the lungs in which gas exchange occurs), while chronic bronchitis affects the bronchi and bronchioles.

## COPD SYMPTOMS

Emphysema and other types of COPD share a number of primary symptoms. If you are experiencing any of the following symptoms, see your doctor. The main symptoms of COPD could also indicate problems other than COPD, and it is important to get an accurate diagnosis.

### Shortness of Breath
Shortness of breath, or dyspnea, may occur as a result of exertion, but may also happen while a person is at rest. In COPD, dyspnea commonly occurs as a result of decreased elasticity of the lungs.

### Cough
A cough is a normal protective reflex that can be brought on by a number of causes, including mechanical or chemical irritation or inflammatory fac-

tors. A cough is the most common symptom of respiratory disease and a prominent sign of chronic bronchitis. An unexplainable cough lasting longer than two or three weeks definitely warrants a visit to your physician.

### Excessive Mucus

Excessive mucus (also known as sputum) that gradually increases over the years is a hallmark of chronic bronchitis and bronchiectasis. Yellow sputum indicates the presence of infection. Green sputum, which suggests the presence of stagnant pus and may be foul-smelling, is commonly associated with bronchiectasis.

### Coughing Up Blood

Coughing up blood from the respiratory tract (hemoptysis) can indicate very serious problems. Causes of coughing up blood include pneumonia, bronchiectasis, tuberculosis, and lung cancer. If you have blood in your sputum, see your physician at once.

### Chest Pain

Chest pain can have myriad causes, but when it relates to respiratory disease, it is often due to inflammation of the parietal pleura (one of the membranes that line the walls of the chest cavity). In any case, chest pain should always be evaluated by a physician.

### Cyanosis

Cyanosis describes a condition in which the skin and mucous membranes (mainly on the face, lips, and earlobes) assume a bluish tinge because there is not enough oxygen in the blood.

### Digital Clubbing

Digital clubbing is a phenomenon in which the fingers take on a drumstick appearance, with slightly enlarged fingertips. The cause of digital clubbing is not understood, but it has been clearly established that approximately 75 percent of digital clubbing is related to respiratory disease, although not necessarily COPD.

## THE ROLE OF INFLAMMATION IN COPD

Inflammation—characterized by the recruitment of white blood cells to the affected area—is part of the immune system's normal response to protect the body against injury and infection.

Inflammation can be acute (occurring immediately in response to an infection or injury) or chronic (long term or ongoing). Chronic (long-term) inflammation is a significant component of chronic bronchitis and bronchiectasis, and may play a role in emphysema as well.

An acute inflammatory reaction is a sign of the immune system's initial response to an invading infection or toxic agent. When the body is subjected to such an insult, the immune system summons white blood cells to protect the affected tissue. Under normal circumstances, the immune system fights the invader and heals the tissue, the acute inflammatory response ceases, and the body reabsorbs the white blood cells. However, if the insult continues or there is a problem with the healing process, the inflammatory response does not cease. White blood cells continue to maintain their presence in the affected tissue, and the acute inflammation eventually progresses to chronic inflammation.

Several types of white blood cells, as well as many other molecules that act as mediators (messengers), are involved in the inflammatory process. (A messenger molecule is a compound that enables one cell to communicate with another cell.) There are a variety of ways in which cells can communicate with one another throughout the body. Some cells release messenger molecules that must travel some distance in the bloodstream before reaching their target cells. Other cells produce messengers that do not enter the blood circulation, but rather exert their action locally, on the cells situated in their immediate area.

Some of the main white blood cells involved in the inflammatory process associated with COPD are lymphocytes, eosinophils, macrophages, and neutrophils. Some of the major classes of mediator molecules that act as messengers between these cells are eicosanoids, cytokines, and chemokines.

The eicosanoids are a major group of local-acting messenger molecules. They are important in regulating the inflammatory response as well as blood clotting, vasoconstriction (narrowing of the veins), vasodilation (expansion of the veins), and bronchoconstriction (narrowing of the bronchioles). The eicosanoid group consists of messenger molecules called leukotrienes, prostaglandins, prostacyclins, and thromboxanes.

A group of leukotrienes called series-4 leukotrienes plays a particularly significant role in COPD. Leukotriene B4 ($LTB_4$) contributes to chronic inflammation in the walls of the bronchi and bronchioles. This pro-inflammatory eicosanoid sends chemical messages to attract leukocytes to the bronchial walls, perpetuating the cycle of chronic inflammation. A number of other series-4 leukotrienes ($LTC_4$, $LTD_4$, and $LTE_4$) are also problematic for people with COPD. These leukotrienes induce the contraction of smooth muscle in the lungs, causing bronchoconstriction.

The body produces these series-4 leukotrienes using a precursor (building-block molecule) known as arachidonic acid. The body obtains arachidonic acid in two ways. The vast majority of the body's arachidonic acid supply comes from dietary sources, mainly animal products such as red meat and dairy foods. The body also creates arachidonic acid through a biochemical reaction in which it converts linoleic acid (an omega-6 essential fatty acid found in the cell membrane) into arachidonic acid.

Arachidonic acid is an omega-6 polyunsaturated fatty acid that is present in the membranes of the body's cells, especially in the brain. Besides being a structural component of cell membranes, it is the precursor to the production of the eicosanoids. It gets converted into the eicosanoids through a complicated series of reactions that use enzymes, including cyclooxygenase, lipoxygenase, and peroxidase. The brain is 60 percent structural lipid, which universally uses arachidonic acid and docosahexaenoic acid (DHA) for growth, function, and structural integrity. Both acids are consistent components of human milk. Moderate amounts of arachidonic acid are necessary for normal brain development and function, especially for infants, but excess arachidonic acid is a major culprit in chronic inflammation.

Arachidonic acid is stored in cell membranes. It is released from a cell membrane and enters into the interior portion of the cell (the cytoplasm) through the action of an enzyme called phospholipase $A_2$. As we shall see in coming chapters, the body's formation of arachidonic acid can be controlled by eating right (for example, cutting down on red meat consumption).

### Chronic Inflammation

Chronic inflammation does not always arise from acute inflammation; it may develop "silently" without any apparent symptoms. This is how the chronic inflammation associated with chronic bronchitis is believed to develop. In many cases of chronic bronchitis, low-grade yet active inflammation is a consequence of constant irritation from cigarette smoke. The inflammatory response starts early in a person's cigarette-smoking history, and as the years go by, the cigarette smoke continues to irritate the cells lining the respiratory tract. This causes an ongoing recruitment of white blood cells to the area, furthering the process of chronic inflammation.

Recurring respiratory infections also contribute to chronic inflammation by further promoting the recruitment of white blood cells to the respiratory tract. White blood cells can also perpetuate their own presence by means of molecular messengers. Activated lymphocytes, for example, release cytokines (messenger molecules) that in turn stimulate macrophages (another kind of immune cell). Stimulated macrophages in turn release different cytokines that activate more lymphocytes.

The continuous presence of white blood cells in the bronchial walls that characterizes chronic inflammation eventually creates myriad problems in the respiratory tract, including edema (swelling) and fibrosis (the formation of excess fibrous connective tissue) in the area around the bronchi and bronchioles. Chronic inflammation can also cause necrosis (tissue death). It is also not clear how chronic inflammation is related to the atypical metaplasia and dysplasia (abnormal cell changes) often seen in the lining of the respiratory tract in people diagnosed with chronic bronchitis. However, it is clear that people who have atypical metaplasia or dysplasia of cells in their respiratory tract are at higher risk for developing lung cancer.

## UNDERSTANDING CHRONIC BRONCHITIS

Bronchitis is defined as inflammation of the bronchial tubes. Chronic bronchitis is recurrent or ongoing bronchitis. The condition is characterized by the excess production of mucus in the bronchi along with a productive cough (a cough that brings up mucus). For a diagnosis of chronic bronchitis, the symptoms must be present on most days for at least three months a year over a period of two consecutive years. Chronic inflammation is a significant component of the overall picture.

The main cause of chronic bronchitis is cigarette smoking, although it can also be caused by inhalation of other toxic substances as well as recurrent respiratory infections. Continuous irritation from cigarette smoke leads to chronic inflammation as well as changes in the physical structure of the mucus-secreting cells and glands lining the respiratory tract. Repeated exposure to the irritating chemical toxins in cigarette smoke causes enlargement (hypertrophy) of the mucus-secreting glands. It also causes an increase in the number of mucus-secreting glands (hyperplasia). You essentially end up with an overabundance of larger-than-normal mucus-secreting glands, which results in oversecretion of mucus into the airway. This excess mucus clogs the airway, often in the form of mucus plugs, and the mucus itself becomes an obstruction in the airway. Cigarette smoke also impairs the sweeping motion of the cilia found on the respiratory epithelium. This contributes further to the obstruction problem as the bronchial passages, which are now faced with even more mucus, are less able to clear themselves.

Evidence also suggests that chronic inflammatory changes occur in the smaller airways, mainly the secondary and tertiary bronchi, and the portion of the bronchioles that contains mucus-secreting cells. As chronic bronchitis and the accompanying inflammation persist, there is a consequent increase in the number of mucus-secreting cells found in these smaller airways, leading to even more mucus production and obstruction of the smaller airways.

Besides obstructing the airways, excess mucus also serves as a breeding ground for bacterial growth. This is one of the main reasons people with COPD so often experience recurrent respiratory infections. Acute episodes of infection are accompanied by inflammation and further mucus production, which make for a vicious cycle that becomes increasingly difficult to manage as COPD progresses.

Although oversecretion of mucus and preventing infection are areas of great concern, the most important issue to address is the underlying inflammation caused by the constant irritation from cigarette smoke or recurrent infections. Treating excess mucus secretion and exacerbations (sudden worsening of symptoms) due to infection will remain an uphill battle if the underlying inflammation is not also addressed.

## UNDERSTANDING EMPHYSEMA

Emphysema is defined as the abnormal and permanent enlargement of the alveoli (airspaces). The central issue in emphysema is collapse of the alveolar walls, which leads to enlargement of the airspaces. The predominant symptom of emphysema is shortness of breath. The onset of shortness of breath occurs early in the development of the disease, and it can become severe as time progresses if measures are not taken to avoid irritants such as smoking and implementing natural health protocols to halt the further destruction of lung tissue.

Collapse of the alveolar walls is caused by the destruction of elastin fibers contained within the walls. (Elastin is a protein, similar in some ways to collagen, that is found in parts of the body such as arteries, lung tissue, skin, and the bladder.) The collapse of these walls results in a loss of surface area for the exchange of carbon dioxide and oxygen, resulting in a significant overall compromise of the process of gas exchange. Destruction of elastin fibers in the alveolar walls also causes the lungs to lose elasticity, affecting their ability to expand and contract.

To help you better visualize what happens to the lungs when the alveolar walls collapse, picture a building full of empty rooms with no windows. Imagine entering the building and immediately heading down a single main hallway. This main hallway represents a respiratory bronchiole. There are a few rooms (alveoli) along this hallway, all of which have an archway opening, with no door attached. Now you take a turn and go down a secondary hallway. This secondary hallway represents an alveolar duct, and there are numerous rooms along this hallway. None of these rooms has a door either, only an archway where a door would be.

Imagine that as you enter any particular room in this secondary hallway, you find another archway in that room that leads to yet another room. Imagine this pattern continuing on to eventually create an elaborate labyrinth. This labyrinth is synonymous with an alveolar sac; the rooms that are interconnected by archways within the labyrinth are the alveoli; and the internal archways themselves are the pores of Kohn (the "holes" between the alveoli). Each one of the initial doorways in the secondary hallway (alveolar duct) leads to its own labyrinth of rooms (alveolar sacs).

Imagine that in any one particular labyrinth (alveolar sac) there are twenty rooms (twenty alveoli) interconnected by archways (pores of Kohn). The archways connect the rooms, and the walls separate the rooms from each other. The surface of the walls (the sheetrock) represents the alveolar wall and the inside of the walls (the studs, plumbing, and so on) represents the interalveolar septum. The studs within the walls represent the matrix of collagen and elastin fibers that makes up the interalveolar septum, and the plumbing represents its capillary network.

Remember that in our building metaphor, the hallways and rooms are all empty; their only purpose is to facilitate the circulation of air. As air travels down the main hallway (the respiratory bronchiole) into the secondary hallway (the alveolar duct), the air is ultimately circulated throughout the rooms (alveoli) as well. As long as clean air is the only thing circulated throughout this system, all is well. When you start circulating cigarette smoke or other noxious substances throughout the system, you begin to have problems. Over time the chemicals in the smoke will wear down the walls, and eventually the walls will collapse and break.

Each "room" in our building has a surface area, which represents the area available for gas exchange. The sum of the surface areas of all the rooms within any particular labyrinth gives us the total surface area

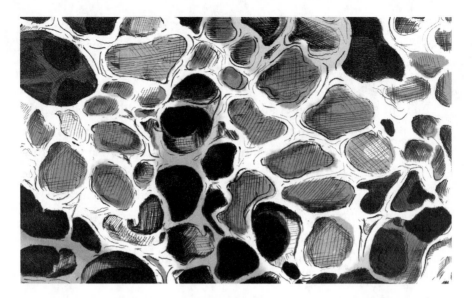

Fig. 5. Normal alveoli. The grayish regions are the alveoli; the darker regions are the alveolar ducts. The thicker white areas within the grayish regions are the interalveolar septa, which serve as the borders, or walls, that separate the alveoli.

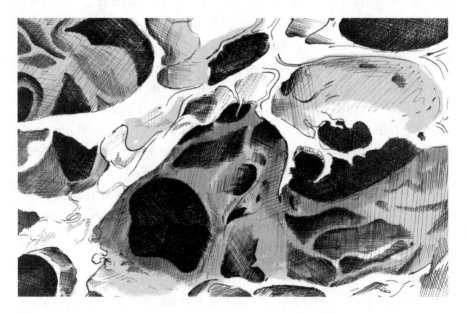

Fig. 6. Alveoli affected by emphysema. Note the enlarged spaces due to the destruction of the alveolar walls.

of that labyrinth. When a wall is destroyed, the surface area of that wall is lost. Instead of having two rooms separated by a wall, there is now just one big room without a dividing wall (in other words, a permanently enlarged airspace). When this damage happens in multiple rooms throughout the labyrinth, you have a serious problem because now many rooms (airspaces) have been enlarged, resulting in a significant overall compromise of the surface area available for gas exchange.

Destruction of the walls of the alveoli also disrupts other structural arrangements in the lungs that are necessary to maintain open, unobstructed airways (mainly the terminal and respiratory bronchioles). Once the structure is disrupted, the lung tissue surrounding the bronchioles is less effective in keeping the airway (bronchiole) open.

Pulmonary fibrosis—overgrowth of fibrous connective tissue, which causes scarring and thickening of the tissue between the air sacs—is a separate and distinct condition from COPD and usually does not occur with emphysema. However, there may be scar tissue in the connective tissue of the lungs as a consequence of inflammation, which is often an ongoing problem for people with COPD. Scar tissue may also be caused by bronchopneumonia, a type of bacterial pneumonia that affects the lungs.

## WHAT CAUSES EMPHYSEMA?

More than 80 percent of all emphysema cases are directly related to cigarette smoking. Ten percent to 15 percent of cases are not smoking related. In these cases, COPD results either from long-term exposure to noxious irritants other than cigarette smoke or alpha-1 antitrypsin (alpha-1 AT) deficiency. Two percent to 5 percent of cases of emphysema are caused by alpha-1 AT deficiency.

Although cigarette smoking is the most common cause of emphysema, other inhaled substances can also produce the condition. Exactly how inhaled noxious chemicals destroy the alveolar wall is still not yet completely understood and remains an area of current research. However, researchers presently believe that the collapse of the alveolar wall is due to a chemical imbalance that causes destruction of the elastin fibers in the alveolar wall, in the area specifically known as the interalveolar septum.

Chemicals in cigarette smoke appear to stimulate the accumulation in the lung of immune cells called macrophages and neutrophils. Nicotine itself attracts neutrophils, and the very presence of nicotine will cause increased recruitment of neutrophils into the lungs. This excessive recruitment of neutrophils into the lungs creates an imbalance that leads to the destruction of the interalveolar septum.

Once in the interalveolar septum, neutrophils release enzymes that in turn degrade proteins. Specifically, in this case, neutrophils release an enzyme called lysosomal elastase, which is very capable of digesting the elastin in the interalveolar septum. Both macrophages and neutrophils release elastase, but neutrophil lysosomal elastase plays a more important role in the destruction of elastin in the alveolar wall. Neutrophil elastase also destroys type IV collagen, another important molecule that contributes to the structure of the alveolar wall.

Neutrophils and alveolar macrophages release a messenger molecule known as leukotriene $B_4$, and leukotriene $B_4$ acts as a signal to recruit more neutrophils. This contributes to the inflammation and destruction of the interalveolar septum.

## The Role of Alpha-1 Antitrypsin

Alpha-1 antitrypsin, known as alpha-1 AT, is a protein made predominantly by the cells of the liver and then released into the blood circulation. One of the purposes of alpha-1 AT is to inhibit the effects of neutrophil elastase in order to keep it from destroying elastin in the alveolar wall. (Elastin, you'll recall, is the principle component of the elastic fibers within the alvelolar wall or interalveolar septum, the membrane that separates the alveoli from one another.)

Under normal circumstances (in the absence of repeated exposure to cigarette smoke or other noxious chemicals), alpha-1 AT diffuses from the capillary circulation into the interalveolar septum to keep the activity of neutrophil elastase at bay. The problem, though, is that cigarette smoke and stimulated neutrophils also release oxygen free radicals. Oxygen free radicals inhibit the activity of alpha-1 AT, rendering it unable to keep neutrophil elastase in check. With alpha-1 AT "tied up" by free radicals, it is unable to stop neutrophil elastase from destroying the elastin within the alveolar wall.

## Alpha-1 AT Deficiency

Because of a genetic (inherited) predisposition, some people may be prone to developing emphysema because their bodies do not correctly make alpha-1 AT. Only 2 percent to 5 percent of cases of emphysema are caused by alpha-1 AT deficiency.

Proteins, including alpha-1 AT, are made up of molecules called amino acids. Amino acids are a collection of about twenty different molecules that, when assembled together into very specific arrangements, become functional proteins. The body itself produces some of these amino acids, but must derive others through food. When you eat foods containing protein, the body digests the protein and breaks it up into amino acid components. The cells of the body then must arrange and assemble those amino acid components in specific sequences for them to become functional proteins that the body can utilize.

In order for alpha-1 AT to be made properly, a series of amino acids must be assembled in a very specific sequence. For various reasons, including genetic inheritance, the sequence can become altered (mutated) so that the alpha-1 AT does not have the ability to perform its normal function: inhibiting the activity of neutrophil elastase.

If you have a genetically inherited alpha-1 AT deficiency, you are at much greater risk for developing emphysema. However, the evidence strongly indicates that even for individuals who have a genetic alpha-1 AT deficiency, cigarette smoking remains the single most important cofactor in the actual development of emphysema. What this means is that if you are alpha-1 AT deficient and you never smoke cigarettes, you may not develop emphysema. If you have a genetically inherited alpha-1 AT deficiency and you do smoke cigarettes, you will in all likelihood develop emphysema. What's more, you will likely also develop it at a much earlier age and experience it much more severely than people who are not alpha-1 AT deficient.

Besides not being able to adequately inhibit neutrophil elastase in the alveolar wall, improperly made alpha-1 AT can cause other significant problems. Aberrant alpha-1 AT can become trapped in the cells of the liver. In adults, the aberrant alpha-1 AT that remains in the liver can lead to cirrhosis of the liver. Alpha-1 AT deficiency rarely ever leads to emphysema in children, but many children affected by alpha-1 AT deficiency develop chronic liver disease, ranging from infant hepatitis to cirrhosis. For these reasons, anyone with alpha-1 AT deficiency should, at a minimum, be taking milk thistle seed extract daily. Milk thistle is an herb that has been very well researched for its ability to protect and support liver function. (See chapter 6 for more information.)

Alpha-1 AT deficiency can be diagnosed with a simple blood test. Anyone who has a history of cigarette smoking should be tested for it. Nonsmokers who begin to develop symptoms that are part of the classic picture for COPD should also be tested. Alpha-1 AT deficiency is treated with weekly intravenous administration of alpha-1 AT derived from human blood. Currently this treatment is available only to patients who meet the criteria of having low enough blood levels of alpha-1 AT and fully manifested emphysema.

## TYPES OF EMPHYSEMA

The precise location along the acinus of the collapsed alveolar walls is largely the determining factor in identifying what type of emphysema a person has. There are four major types of emphysema.

Bullae are enlarged airspaces that are greater than 1 cm (a little less than half an inch) in diameter and can be present with any of the four types of emphysema. They occupy areas right next to the visceral pleura, usually near the apex (top) of the lungs. When these localized areas are especially prominent, the condition is sometimes referred to as bullous emphysema. Bullous emphysema presents its own unique set of concerns due to the potential size of the bullae and their potential for rupture.

## Summary of the Sequence of Events in the Destruction of the Alveolar Wall

1. The acinus is repeatedly exposed to cigarette smoke or other noxious chemicals.

2. Continuous exposure to smoke or toxins induces excessive recruitment of macrophages and neutrophils into the lung. Macrophages release neutrophil chemotactic factors (attractants), which attract neutrophils into the lung. Nicotine itself is a chemotactic, or attracting agent, for neutrophils, so it also attracts neutrophils into the lung.

3. Upon entering the lung, neutrophils escape capillary circulation and find their way into the interalveolar septum.

4. Once in the interalveolar septum, neutrophils release lysosomal elastase, an enzyme that degrades elastin, the principal component of the elastic fibers within the interalveolar septum. Neutrophils can also perpetuate their own existence through their release of the molecular messenger leukotriene $B_4$.

5. Alpha-1 antitrypsin, a protein that would normally inhibit the action of neutrophil elastase, is rendered ineffective due to being tied up by reactive oxygen free radicals released from neutrophils as well as oxidants in cigarette smoke.

6. As a result of elastin in the interalveolar septum being degraded by neutrophil elastase, the alveolar wall collapses, resulting in permanent, abnormal enlargement of the airspaces and a lessening of the elasticity of the lungs.

Bullae that become large enough can compromise breathing by compressing healthy lung tissue next to the bullae. A ruptured bulla can give rise to a condition called spontaneous pneumothorax, in which air or gas enters the space between a lung and the inner chest wall and causes the lung to collapse.

## Centrilobular Emphysema

Centrilobular or centriacinar emphysema is the most common type of emphysema. It involves primarily the respiratory bronchioles and their alveoli. The alveoli within the alveolar sacs are usually less involved. This is the type of emphysema seen most often in cigarette smokers, and it predominantly affects the upper lobes of the lung, in the area of the lung closest to the shoulder. There is usually inflammation in the bronchi, bronchioles, and the interalveolar septum. Because of the strong link with cigarette smoking, this form of emphysema is often seen in combination with chronic bronchitis.

## Panlobular Emphysema

Panlobular or panacinar emphysema is the type of emphysema most often associated with alpha-1 AT deficiency. Panlobular emphysema tends to occur more often in the lower zones of the lung and is most severe at the base of the lung. In panlobular emphysema, the entire acinus is affected, and uniform enlargement of the airspaces is present from the respiratory bronchiole all the way to the distal (farthest) alveoli. In cases of panlobular emphysema where the damage is extensive, there is marked reduction in the gas exchange surface (alveoli–capillary interface) as well as a reduction in the elastic recoil properties of the lungs.

## Paraseptal Emphysema

Paraseptal or distal acinar emphysema affects predominantly the most distal part of the acinus, the alveolar sacs, and alveoli. The emphysema is more severe at the edges of the lobules and in areas near the pleura (the membrane lining the thoracic cavity). It also tends to occur next to areas that have are scarred or affected by fibrosis. This type of emphysema is usually more severe in the upper regions of the lungs and can be the cause of spontaneous pneumothorax.

## Irregular Emphysema

This type of emphysema is associated with scarring in the lungs. It is called irregular emphysema because it can affect any part of the acinus.

## BRONCHIECTASIS

Bronchiectasis is a chronic condition characterized by irreversible dilation (expansion or stretching) and distortion (twisting out of shape) of the bronchi and bronchioles. The airways are abnormally dilated with variable amounts of mucus and inflammation. Normal structural components of the bronchial wall are destroyed and often replaced by fibrous connective tissue. Bronchiectasis is characterized by a chronic, loose, productive cough containing significant amounts of foul-smelling sputum.

The exact cause of bronchiectasis is not clearly understood. Evidence suggests it may occur as a result of recurrent infections, often pneumonia, that cause chronic inflammation. This chronic inflammation weakens the bronchial walls so that they become stretched and twisted from their normal shape and form. Mucus and pus accumulate in these dilated areas, which contributes to the cycle of infection. The recurring infections cause even more damage to the lungs, establishing a vicious cycle that becomes increasingly difficult to manage.

Although the cause of bronchiectasis may not be directly related to cigarette smoking, bronchiectasis is often seen in combination with emphysema or chronic bronchitis because it is also related to chronic infection and inflammation. The recurrent infections characteristic of chronic bronchitis can exacerbate any existing bronchiectasis. Therefore, as with chronic bronchitis, the main issue in treating bronchiectasis is to reduce inflammation as much as possible. By reducing inflammation, less mucus will be produced, and with less mucus, there will be less chance of infection. Less mucus will also result in a less obstructed airway, so breathing will be easier.

As we have seen, COPD is the blanket term that traditionally encompasses emphysema, chronic bronchitis, and bronchiectasis. Emphysema and chronic bronchitis have a number of common symptoms because

TABLE 3.

COMPARISON OF EMPHYSEMA AND CHRONIC BRONCHITIS

|  | Emphysema | Chronic Bronchitis |
|---|---|---|
| Location | Acinus | Bronchi and bronchioles |
| Major cause | Tobacco smoke | Tobacco smoke, inhaled irritants, recurrent infections |
| Clinical changes | Enlargement of airspaces; alveolar wall destruction | Hyperplasia and hypertrophy of mucus glands in respiratory tract |
| Major symptom | Dyspnea | Cough with sputum |
| Dyspnea | Severe, early onset | Mild, late onset |
| Cough/sputum | Occurring late in the progression of disease, with slight sputum | Occurring early, with a great deal of sputum |
| Elastic recoil | Greatly reduced | Normal |
| Airway resistance | Normal, slightly increased | Increased |
| Infection | Occasional | Common |
| Lung volume* | Decreased $FEV_1$, increased TLC and RV | Decreased $FEV_1$, normal TLC, slight RV increase |
| Body appearance | Thin, asthenic | Strong, adequately nourished |
| Cyanosis | Rare | Common |

*See pages 43–44 for explanations of these tests for measuring lung volume.

people often have varying degrees of both of these conditions. Shortness of breath, a productive cough, and increased susceptibility to infections are all common features of emphysema and chronic bronchitis, and the severity of any of these symptoms is dependent upon which condition is predominant.

Should you have any of the symptoms or issues that have been discussed in this chapter, it is important for you to see a doctor and obtain a proper diagnosis to ascertain what is going on with your body. This is especially true for those of you who are experiencing these symptoms and have an extensive history of cigarette smoking. You may already suspect that you have COPD because these symptoms have been progressing over the years. I urge you not to hesitate any longer in seeing your doctor. Doing so now and obtaining an appropriate diagnosis can be a positive starting point for you to turn your health around.

# 3

# Diagnosis and Conventional Treatment of COPD

COPD ordinarily develops over the course of many years. A diagnosis is usually made when symptoms become problematic, leading a physician to order additional tests. A patient's medical history, physical examination, test results, and radiographic studies can indicate with a high degree of probability the presence of emphysema, but there is no way to determine the exact amount of damage in a living person. Fortunately, however, it is not necessary to know the precise type of emphysema a person has or the amount of damage present in order to proceed with treatment.

## DIAGNOSTIC TESTS FOR COPD

In order to evaluate your symptoms, your physician will need to study your past medical history and conduct a thorough physical examination. He or she will also probably order various blood tests and other diagnostic procedures to confirm the diagnosis of COPD. Some of the tests or procedures that may be used to confirm COPD are as follows.

### Radiological Procedures
Radiological procedures include chest x-rays and CT scans. The chest x-ray is often used to rule out any other lung diseases besides COPD

such as pneumonia and lung cancer—the chest x-ray itself is often imprecise in determining whether or not a person has COPD, unless the COPD is quite severe. A CT scan may provide more accuracy in diagnosing COPD, although some abnormal lung anatomy still may not be detected. In individuals who are predominantly affected with emphysema, the chest x-ray may show an enlarged chest cavity along with decreased lung markings that reflect damaged lung tissue and enlargement of the airspaces (alveoli). In individuals who are predominantly affected with chronic bronchitis, the chest x-ray may show increased lung markings, which represent the thickened, inflamed, and scarred airways. A CT scan of the chest is a specialized x-ray that can reveal the abnormal lung tissue and airways in COPD with reasonable accuracy.

### Arterial Blood Gas Tests

Arterial blood yields very useful information that cannot be obtained from venous blood. Arterial blood is measured to determine $PaO_2$ (the partial pressure of oxygen, or the concentration of oxygen in the arterial blood), $SaO_2$ (the percentage of hemoglobin saturated with oxygen in the arterial blood), and $PaCO_2$ (the partial pressure of carbon dioxide, or the concentration of carbon dioxide in the arterial blood). Arterial blood gas testing is also used to determine the pH (acidity) of the blood. Arterial blood gases for testing are usually obtained from blood drawn from an artery in the wrist.

Abnormally low values of $PaO_2$ indicate hypoxemia (inadequate levels of oxygen in the blood) and also often indicate hypoxia (inadequate amounts of oxygen reaching the tissues). Elevated values of $PaCO_2$ indicate a state known as hypercapnia, which may affect people with COPD because they tend to retain carbon dioxide. This is an area of particular concern, as people with COPD can become so tolerant of the elevated carbon dioxide levels that hypoxia becomes the principal drive for respiration. Under these circumstances, if the patient is receiving supplemental oxygen, the amount of oxygen being given must be carefully controlled. If the person receives too high a concentration of oxygen, a proportionate amount of carbon dioxide will be produced, but the carbon dioxide will be retained due to decreased ability to ventilate. The retained carbon dioxide can cause a very serious condition called respiratory acidosis, indicated by a marked lowering of the pH of the blood (increased acidity of the blood).

## Oximetry

Oximetry, commonly called pulse ox, is another test to measure the amount of oxygen in the blood. The measurement is made via a plastic clip placed on the fingertip in the hospital or the doctor's office. The information it provides is not as accurate as the information derived from an arterial blood gas test. However, the test is practical in that it can be used to measure the oxygenation of the blood during activity or during sleep.

## Alpha-1 Antitrypsin Level Test

This is a simple blood test to determine if you have the genetically inherited form of emphysema due to an alpha-1 AT deficiency.

## Pulmonary Function Tests

In general, there are four aspects to pulmonary function testing. They are spirometry, post-bronchodilator spirometry, lung volume testing, and diffusion capacity.

### SPIROMETRY

This test measures the amount of air entering and exiting the lungs and is the most reliable way of assessing reversible airway obstruction. To perform the test, the patient first inhales as deeply as possible and then exhales as forcefully and rapidly as possible into the spirometry machine, until he can exhale no more. This is called "forced exhalation." The test yields several measurements. The measurements most useful for determining the presence of COPD are the forced expiratory volume after one second ($FEV_1$) and the forced vital capacity (FVC).

People with COPD typically show a reduction in the amount of air exhaled (FVC) compared with individuals with healthy lungs. Those with COPD also show a reduction in the amount of air exhaled during the initial first second of exhalation (FEV$_1$), and the degree of reduction in FEV$_1$ is greater than the FVC reduction. This means that people with COPD not only exhale less, but they also exhale significantly less during the first second of exhalation. Individuals with healthy lungs usually exhale about 75 percent of the air they inhaled during the first second of exhalation.

### POST-BRONCHODILATOR SPIROMETRY

Post-bronchodilator spirometry utilizes the same process that is used for regular spirometry, except that it is performed after the patient has been given a bronchodilator drug, such as albuterol. If there is improvement in the FEV$_1$ after this test, it indicates that the airways are responsive to the drug and that it may be useful in the management of the airway obstruction.

### LUNG VOLUME TESTING

Lung volume testing reveals very useful information in the diagnosis of emphysema. Two important measurements obtained from lung volume testing are residual volume (RV) and total lung capacity (TLC). A high TLC indicates hyperinflation (overinflation) of the lungs and a high RV indicates that air is being trapped in the lungs. High values for TLC and RV suggest that the patient has emphysema.

### DIFFUSION CAPACITY

This test measures how much gas is transferred from the alveoli into the capillaries. For the test, the patient inhales a very small, safe amount of carbon monoxide and then the blood is tested to see how much carbon monoxide diffused from the lungs into the bloodstream. A reduced diffusion capacity suggests that the patient may have emphysema. Table 4 (see page 44) provides a summary of the abbreviations used in some of the various diagnostic tests for COPD.

## TABLE 4. MEANING OF ABBREVIATIONS USED
## IN DIAGNOSTIC TESTS FOR COPD

| | |
|---|---|
| $PaO_2$ | The partial pressure (concentration) of oxygen in arterial blood. |
| $SaO_2$ | The percentage of hemoglobin saturated with oxygen in arterial blood. |
| $PaCO_2$ | The partial pressure (concentration) of carbon dioxide in arterial blood. |
| $FEV_1$ | Forced expiratory volume in one second. This is the amount of air exhaled in one second after maximal inhalation. |
| FVC | Forced vital capacity. This is the maximal amount of air exhaled after maximal inhalation. |
| RV | Residual volume. This is the amount of air left in the lungs after a forced exhalation. |
| TLC | Total lung capacity. This is the amount of air that can be contained in the lungs after maximal inhalation. |
| DLCO | Diffusion capacity of the lungs for carbon monoxide. |

## CONVENTIONAL TREATMENTS FOR COPD

The main goal of conventional medicine in the treatment of COPD is to manage symptoms, usually with pharmaceutical drugs. While some of these drugs are absolutely necessary to help certain people with COPD keep breathing, they will not provide any benefit in terms of restorative healing. The good news is that you can get started with the nutritional and natural health therapies discussed in this book while remaining on your current COPD medications. However, you should always consult with your physician before implementing any alternative treatment strategies. If your current doctor is unable or unwilling to support your choice to utilize nutritional and other natural treatments, appendix 1 provides a list of organizations that can help you find another physician or qualified health care provider experienced with alternative or integrative medicine.

Depending upon the severity of your condition, you may find that if you are faithful to the dietary changes and other natural health strategies discussed in this book, you may very well end up needing less of your pharmaceutical medications. You might even improve so much that you can stop taking them altogether. However, it is important not to stop or change the dosage of your pharmaceutical medications without the advice and guidance of your doctor. Always consult with your physician before you stop taking or reduce the dosage of any prescribed medications.

The following are the most commonly prescribed types of medications used in the treatment of COPD.

## Bronchodilators

Bronchodilators are drugs prescribed to promote the relaxation of the smooth muscle that surrounds the bronchi and bronchioles. With the relaxation of bronchial smooth muscle, the bronchi and bronchioles can expand and allow for improved airflow. Bronchodilators are classified into three major categories:

1. Short-acting and long-acting beta-2 agonists
2. Anticholinergic agents
3. Methylxanthines

### BETA-2 AGONISTS

Short-acting beta-2 agonists include albuterol, metaproterenol, terbutaline, and pirbuterol. These drugs produce a maximum amount of bronchodilation 5 to 15 minutes after they are taken and continue to act for 4 to 6 hours. Long-acting beta-2 agonists include salmeterol and oral sustained-release albuterol. These drugs produce bronchodilation after 15 to 30 minutes and can last up to 12 hours.

### ANTICHOLINERGIC AGENTS

This group of drugs includes ipratropium bromide and tiotropium bromide. These drugs induce relaxation of the smooth muscle surrounding the bronchi by blocking muscarinic receptor sites, preventing stimulation that would cause bronchoconstriction. Muscarinic receptors are receptors on the smooth muscle that surrounds the bronchi. These receptors are stimulated by acetylcholine, a neurotransmitter, or messenger chemical, produced by the body. When the receptors are stimulated by acetylcholine, the smooth muscle contracts, thereby inducing bronchoconstriction. By binding to the receptor, ipratropium bromide blocks acetylcholine from binding and thus keeps the smooth muscle in a relaxed state. Ipratropium acts within 30 to 60 minutes and can last up to 6 hours. Tiotropium also begins to act within 30 to 60 minutes but can last up to 24 hours.

## METHYLXANTHINES

The agent most commonly used for COPD in this group is theophylline. The mechanism of action of theophylline is not fully understood, but it is believed to help ease breathing by promoting the relaxation of bronchial smooth muscle. Theophylline is taken orally usually once or twice a day. Rapid-acting theophylline peaks in 1 to 2 hours and lasts up to 6 hours. Delayed-acting theophylline peaks in about 4 to 8 hours and lasts 8 to 24 hours.

## Corticosteroids

Corticosteroid drugs are often prescribed to help reduce the inflammation that is part of COPD. If you have COPD, you are more than likely familiar with prednisone, one of the most commonly prescribed corticosteroids, which is taken orally. There are also a variety of inhaled corticosteroids, such as budesonide, fluticasone, triamcinolone, and flunisonide.

Prednisone is often prescribed for people with COPD when inflammation is particularly severe. In my opinion, prednisone should be used only as a very last resort because of its dangerous and damaging side effects. Prednisone effectively reduces inflammation by inhibiting phospholipase $A_2$. Inhibition of phospholipase $A_2$ inhibits the release of arachidonic acid from the cell membrane, which impairs the production of pro-inflammatory eicosanoids. This is a powerful way to reduce inflammation, but prednisone has many dangerous side effects:

1. Sodium retention (this raises blood pressure as well as increases the viscosity of mucus secretions)
2. Increased fat deposits
3. Increased stomach acidity
4. Increased sweating, especially at night
5. Hyperglycemia (elevated blood sugar levels)
6. Photosensitivity (increased sensitivity to the sun)
7. Decreased ability to fight infection (immune suppression)
8. Thrush (growth of the fungus *Candida albicans* in the mouth and throat)
9. Bone, muscle, and eye problems
10. Acne on the face, back, and chest
11. Delayed wound healing
12. Vulnerability to depression
13. Nausea, vomiting, and peptic ulcers
14. Suppression of adrenal gland function
15. Cataracts and increased intraocular pressure

### Expectorant and Mucolytic Medications

Expectorants and mucolytics are prescribed for their ability to help thin mucus secretions and move them out of the airway. Guaifenesin is one commonly prescribed expectorant; it is also now available over the counter under the brand name Mucinex in 600 mg extended-release tablets. Acetylcysteine is a commonly prescribed mucolytic substance that is discussed in detail in chapter 6, because acetylcysteine is also available as a nutritional supplement. The prescription form of acetylcysteine is a liquid that you use in a nebulizer. The nonprescription form is called N-acetylcysteine, or NAC, and comes in capsule form.

### Antibiotics

Antibiotics are prescribed to kill disease-causing bacteria during the acute stage of an infection. Because many people with COPD have recurrent or chronic respiratory tract infections, they may undergo multiple courses of treatment with antibiotics. This can lead to antibiotic resistance, meaning the antibiotics become less effective at killing the bacteria over time. Antibiotic resistance is a growing problem in hospitals and can also lead to complications in the treatment of COPD-related infections.

## Physical and Respiratory Therapy

Physical therapy and respiratory therapy are a collection of therapeutic methods that have common goals of helping to eliminate mucus from the respiratory tract, enhance the efficiency of breathing, and strengthen respiratory muscles. These therapies are usually performed by a physical or respiratory therapist or a family member who has been specially trained.

Specific physical therapies for the lungs include deep-breathing exercises, coughing, turning, postural drainage, cupping (also called percussion), and vibration.

Turning from side to side permits lung expansion. Patients may turn themselves or be turned by a caregiver. Postural drainage uses the force of gravity to assist in effectively draining secretions from the lungs and into the central airway, where they can be either coughed up or suctioned out. The patient is placed in a head- or chest-down position and is kept in this position for up to 15 minutes.

Cupping is rhythmically striking the chest wall with cupped hands. The purpose of this percussion is to break up thick secretions in the lungs so that they can be more easily removed. Percussion is performed on each lung segment for 1 to 2 minutes at a time.

In similar fashion to percussion, the purpose of vibration is to help break up lung secretions. Vibration can be either mechanical or manual. It is performed as the patient breathes deeply. When done manually, the person performing the vibration places his or her hands against the patient's chest and creates vibrations by quickly contracting and relaxing arm and shoulder muscles while the patient exhales. Mechanically it is performed by the patient wearing a vest or jacket that is connected to a machine that forces pulsations of air through the jacket, creating a vibratory effect that helps to loosen mucus.

These physical therapies for the lungs are often performed in conjunction with other respiratory treatments designed to rid the airways of mucus secretions. These may include suctioning, nebulizer treatments, aerosol humidification, and administration of expectorant drugs.

### Surgery

In very serious cases of COPD, there are three procedures that may be considered: lung transplant, lung volume reduction surgery, and bullectomy.

1. Lung transplant is a very invasive procedure that is considered only for extremely severe cases of COPD. Certain specific criteria for $FEV_1$ and $PaCO_2$ must be met in order for a patient to be considered for this surgery.
2. Lung volume reduction involves the surgical removal of seriously damaged portions of the lung. The goal of this surgery is improving the elastic recoil of the remaining lung tissue while at the same time improving airflow and exercise capacity.
3. Bullectomy is the surgical removal of bullae in the lungs. Once the bullae are removed, the healthy air sacs have more room to expand, and the muscles used to breathe can function better.

Because COPD is a serious and potentially life-threatening disease, it is essential that you receive diagnosis and treatment from a qualified health care practitioner. While pharmaceutical drugs may be necessary and even lifesaving in some instances, there are limitations to what drugs can offer someone with COPD. However, as we shall see, natural medicine offers myriad alternatives to help you get control of your symptoms and improve your quality of life.

# Quitting Smoking

If you've been diagnosed with COPD and are still smoking cigarettes, this chapter is for you. In order for your healing process to begin, you must quit smoking cigarettes. In fact, quitting smoking now is the single most important thing you can do for your health.

Many people first receive a diagnosis of COPD when they are in their forties or older, after twenty or more years of smoking. Some people are able to quit smoking right away. Unfortunately, others continue to smoke even after they have been diagnosed with COPD. If you are one of these people, take heart. It is not too late. By the time my father quit smoking, his COPD was quite severe. He did not begin using natural health methods to care for his COPD until the age of sixty-nine. Through a combination of quitting smoking, changing his diet, using herbs and supplements, and adopting other lifestyle changes, he turned his condition around dramatically and had a much improved quality of life until he went to his final rest, at the age of eighty-three.

For most smokers, the thought of quitting is a psychological mine-field. While we know smoking is bad for us, most smokers are power-fully attached to cigarettes. As a veteran smoker (and quitter) myself, I know that many methods for quitting can work, but they're only as good as your resolve to stay off cigarettes. Quitting smoking is an ongoing process that involves positive changes in both mind-set and lifestyle. You can choose to become a nonsmoker and think positively about it.

You may have already tried to quit and failed one or more times. Don't give up. Studies show that many people must attempt to quit a number of times before they finally succeed. I know how difficult quitting smoking is, because I struggled with quitting myself. When I finally quit, it was after about a dozen attempts.

Receiving a diagnosis of COPD in and of itself is going to be enough to enable many of you to quit right away. Others, though, are going to struggle with quitting because the nature of nicotine addiction is complex and powerful. Over the years, smoking has probably attached itself to virtually every aspect of your life, and learning how to disassociate smoking from the events of your daily life is going to take an incredible amount of willpower.

You may wish you could turn back time and never start smoking in the first place. Instead of blaming yourself for your current health problems, try to think positively about the improvements you can bring about in your health.

There are several benefits that you will receive immediately upon quitting or soon after:

- Within thirty minutes of your last cigarette, your blood pressure and your pulse will decrease and the temperature of your hands and feet will increase.
- Eight hours after your last cigarette, the levels of carbon monoxide in your blood will have dropped to normal and the oxygen level in your blood will have increased to normal.
- At twenty-four hours after your last cigarette, your risk of heart attack will have decreased.
- Forty-eight hours after your last cigarette, your nerve endings will begin to regrow and your sense of smell and taste will be enhanced.
- Two weeks to three months after you quit, your circulation will improve, walking will become easier, and your lung function will increase.
- During the first one to nine months after you quit, your coughing,

sinus congestion, shortness of breath, and fatigue will decrease.

- After one year, your risk of coronary heart disease will be reduced to half that of a smoker.

Of course, there are also long-term benefits to quitting smoking.

- From five to fifteen years after quitting smoking, your risk for stroke decreases to that of people who never smoked.
- Ten years after quitting, your risk of lung cancer drops to half that of smokers. The risk of cancers of the mouth, throat, esophagus, bladder, kidney, and pancreas all decrease, and the risk of developing ulcers decreases.
- Fifteen years after quitting, your risk of coronary heart disease is similar to that of those who have never smoked and your risk of death returns to the level of people who have never smoked.

### Cigarettes and COPD

Cigarette smoking is the main cause of COPD for a variety of reasons. Cigarette smoke impairs the sweeping motion of cilia on the respiratory epithelium, which impairs the ability of the bronchi and larger bronchioles to stay clean and free of debris. Cigarette smoke causes hypertrophy (enlargement) and hyperplasia (an increase in number) of the mucus-secreting glands that line the respiratory tract, leading to excess mucus secretion that clogs the airways. Cigarette smoke causes chronic inflammation in the lungs by inducing the continuous recruitment of neutrophils into the lungs. Neutrophils in turn release neutrophil elastase, the enzyme that destroys elastin, which destroys the alveolar wall. Cigarette smoke also interferes with the activity of alpha-1 AT, the protein that protects against the damaging effects of neutrophil elastase. Cigarette smoke causes smooth muscle constriction, increasing airway resistance and making breathing more difficult.

You will not be able to rebuild your health overnight, of course. But by quitting smoking now, you will have taken the first and most important step toward developing a lifestyle that will improve your health and your quality of living for the rest of your life.

## MAKING THE DECISION TO QUIT

Cigarette smoking is a powerful addiction. Nicotine, the addictive substance in tobacco, has been likened to heroin in that it is one of the most physically addictive substances known to humankind. If you smoke, you also have a psychological addiction to the habit of smoking, in that much of your life revolves around cigarettes and smoking. It is only when you try to stop smoking that you become aware of how many aspects of your life are affected by your smoking habit. It may be difficult to even imagine participating in certain activities without having a cigarette. For example, you may be accustomed to having a cigarette after each meal or when you're on the phone. These are times at which your craving for a cigarette may be particularly strong.

Instead of focusing on how difficult it will be to live without cigarettes, begin to envision the benefits of being "smoke-free." For example, in addition to the obvious health benefits and living longer, your clothes and breath will no longer smell bad, and you will no longer be forced to go outside like a pariah to smoke.

You will also save a great deal of money. Most people diagnosed with COPD will have, on average, smoked between 150,000 and 400,000 cigarettes and spent as much as $50,000 on cigarettes at the time of their initial diagnosis.

Here are some additional benefits you can expect to enjoy when you quit smoking:

- Your house and your car will not smell like cigarettes.
- You can get rid of your dirty ashtrays.
- Every breath you take will feel clean and refreshing.

- Your sense of smell will return, and you will be able to taste your food properly again.
- You'll have whiter teeth and fresher breath.
- You'll have more stamina and endurance, and you won't get tired as often during the day.
- You won't have to worry about attending events where you can't smoke.
- Your complexion will improve.
- You'll no longer have to fear causing a fire with your cigarettes.
- You'll no longer have any guilt about exposing family and friends to secondhand smoke.
- Your heart will feel more relaxed, and it will be able do more work with less effort.
- You'll have less heartburn and indigestion, and your coughing will lessen.
- If you have sinus problems or allergies, they will improve.
- Your anxiety level will drop way down, you'll be more in control of yourself, and you'll enjoy sharper thinking.
- You'll have renewed confidence in your ability to achieve whatever goal you set for yourself.

## METHODS TO HELP YOU QUIT SMOKING

Quitting smoking requires tremendous willpower. This means you must have a strong desire to quit smoking and the will to stick to your decision to quit. However, you don't have to go "cold turkey." A variety of methods and programs can help you break the physical addiction to nicotine as well as your psychological attachments to the smoking habit.

Some methods for quitting may prove more useful to you than others. There are a number of techniques designed to help you quit, ranging from counseling to acupuncture to herbs and nicotine replacement therapy. You may find that you need to employ more than one technique in order to achieve your goal of becoming a nonsmoker. If you have tried to quit before but were not successful, this does not mean you are weak-willed. All it means is that either the timing wasn't right or you didn't prepare yourself well enough to meet this formidable challenge with success. Don't give up—your chances for success increase with each successive attempt you make to quit.

Today is a new day and if you really want to quit badly enough, you can still succeed at this. Prepare yourself mentally and emotionally, plan out your course of action, and organize your support resources.

Take the necessary time to understand some of the triggers that provoke your desire to smoke a cigarette. Are there particular people with whom you will want to smoke? Are there certain places that you associate with having a cigarette? Are there certain activities that you associate with smoking—having a drink or a cup of coffee, or being on the phone, or driving your car? Are there particular times that you associate with smoking—after a meal, just before you go to bed, or when you are bored or stressed out? Understanding and recognizing these situations as triggers of your impulse to light up will prepare you to be less vulnerable and strengthen your chances for success as you begin your journey to become a nonsmoker.

## Acupuncture

Acupuncture (the insertion of very thin needles into various points on the body) is widely used in treating addictions. Acupuncture is steadily establishing itself as a very viable alternative in helping smokers to become ex-smokers when it is used as part of a program that also combines other smoking-cessation techniques—such as one-on-one or group counseling, cessation education, and other behavioral training. Acupuncture is not a panacea or a magic cure in the treatment of nicotine addiction; however, it can help to reduce the cravings and lessen the withdrawal symptoms associated with quitting.

An important consideration for the success of acupuncture is the level of preparation and commitment to stop smoking on the part of the patient. When used as part of a smoking-cessation program, acupuncture is aimed at not only relieving the immediate symptoms related to smoking cessation, but also toward restoring imbalances that exist in the body. To that end, acupuncture treatments will always be used holistically in conjunction with Chinese herbs, nutritional modifications, bodywork, and exercise to address the irritability, nervousness, and cravings associated with smoking cessation and to assist with relaxation and detoxification. (For a more detailed discussion of acupuncture, see chapter 9.) Appendix 1 contains information that can help you find a qualified acupuncturist.

### Herbs

There are several herbs with a traditional reputation for helping people quit smoking. These herbs exert varying effects that will ease the process of smoking cessation. Most of them can be found in either dried bulk, capsule, or liquid extract form. Follow the directions on the label for use. If using dried herbs, use them only to prepare tea, and never smoke them as a replacement for tobacco. See appendix 1 for information on how to find a qualified herbalist.

**Lobelia** *(Lobelia inflata):* Lobelia is a very powerful herb that helps to calm the mind and relax the body. It has helped many people to control their cravings for nicotine. Lobelia is also reputed to have the effect of making cigarettes taste very bad. Lobelia is not recommended if you are pregnant or nursing, or for people with high blood pressure or for those prone to faintness. Lobelia may cause nausea and vomiting if too much is taken.

**St. John's wort** *(Hypericum perforatum):* St. John's wort is one of the best known herbs for promoting a positive mental attitude—something people often need help with during the early phases of becoming a non-smoker. St. John's wort can have potentially dangerous interactions with some prescription drugs. Consult your physician before taking St. John's wort if you are currently taking prescription antidepressants, anticoagulants, oral contraceptives, antiseizure medications, drugs to treat HIV or prevent transplant rejection, or any other prescription drug. St. John's wort is not recommended if you are pregnant or nursing.

**Black cohosh** *(Actaea racemosa,* formerly *Cimicifuga racemosa):* Black cohosh is commonly used by women to help them stay balanced during their monthly cycle. However, it is also known to be a safe sedative that relieves nervousness and anxiety, which makes it useful for the irritability, restlessness, and nervousness associated with quitting smoking. Excessive consumption of black cohosh can irritate the nervous system and may cause nausea. Black cohosh is not recommended if you are pregnant or nursing. Avoid black cohosh if you have any heart conditions as large doses can cause low blood pressure. Very large amounts of this herb (more than several grams daily) may cause abdominal pain, headache, and/or dizziness.

**Blue vervain** *(Verbena hastata):* Blue vervain has been referred to as a natural tranquilizer and as such it can be used to calm the nerves. It can also be used for insomnia. There are no known warnings or contraindications for blue vervain.

**Catnip** *(Nepeta cataria):* Catnip has a soothing and relaxing effect on the digestive system, and helps to relieve diarrhea, flatulence, indigestion, upset stomach, and headache. Catnip also has antispasmodic properties that make it useful for abdominal cramps as well as chronic coughing. Catnip is also good for alleviating sleeplessness. Catnip's antibiotic and astringent properties are also beneficial for treating colds and bronchial infections. Catnip has no known warnings or contraindications.

**Hyssop** *(Hyssopus officinalis):* Hyssop is discussed later in the book for its ability to help with clearing mucus congestion in the lungs associated with COPD. It also has been known to alleviate the anxiety and even hysteria that is sometimes associated with smoking withdrawal. Hyssop is not recommended during pregnancy, or if you have epilepsy or high blood pressure.

**Korean ginseng** *(Panax ginseng):* Ginseng is one of the herbs discussed later in the book because of its immense usefulness for COPD, but it is being mentioned here because it can be very helpful in smoking cessation as well. Ginseng is one of the most popular herbs in the world for stimulating energy and helping the body to deal with stress. This property enables ginseng to help alleviate the fatigue and anxiety related to quitting smoking. Ginseng is known to help reestablish balance in the body's systems, which can be helpful to smokers as their bodies adjust to the absence of nicotine. It has been used to help lower cholesterol, balance the metabolism, increase energy levels, and stimulate the immune system. Ginseng also helps to increase oxygenation to the cells and tissues, promotes detoxification, and stimulates the regeneration of damaged cells. Higher than recommended dosages of ginseng taken at bedtime can cause insomnia.

**Motherwort** *(Leonurus cardiaca):* Motherwort is usually used for heart and/or circulation problems or for menstrual and uterine conditions. Motherwort, however, also has properties that enable it to act as a sedative, inducing tranquillity in times of anxiety associated with quitting smoking. Motherwort is not recommended during pregnancy or for those who experience excessive menstrual bleeding.

**Oat straw or oat seed** *(Avena sativa):* In folk medicine, oats were used to treat nervous exhaustion, insomnia, and weakness of the nerves. A tincture of the green tops of oats was also used to help with withdrawal from tobacco addiction. Oats were often used in baths to treat insomnia and anxiety. Oats are one of the best remedies for stress, nervous debility, and exhaustion, especially when associated with depression (a common affliction in people who have recently quit smoking). Oats have no known warnings or contraindications.

**Peppermint** *(Mentha × piperita):* Peppermint is a good herb to have on hand for the digestive complaints, anxiety, and tension issues related to smoking cessation. Peppermint has a relaxing effect on the muscles of the digestive system, combats flatulence, and stimulates the flow of bile and other digestive juices. The volatile oil in peppermint acts as a mild anesthetic to the stomach wall, which helps alleviate feelings of nausea.

Where headaches are associated with digestion, peppermint may help. Peppermint also eases anxiety and tension. Peppermint has no known warnings or contraindications.

**Skullcap** *(Scutellaria lateriflora):* Skullcap contains plant compounds that help the brain produce more endorphins (naturally occurring chemicals that promote feelings of well-being)—this is believed to enhance both awareness and calmness. Skullcap relaxes states of nervous tension while renewing and reviving the central nervous system. It has traditionally been used in combination with valerian (see below) as a mild sedative for anxiety. Skullcap also aids sleep, improves circulation, strengthens the heart, and relieves muscle cramps, pain, spasms, and stress. Skullcap is useful in treating anxiety, fatigue, cardiovascular disease, headache, hyperactivity, and nervousness, and has also shown potential in treating drug addiction. Skullcap is not recommended during pregnancy or if you are nursing.

**Slippery elm** *(Ulmus rubra):* Slippery elm is rich in nutrients and easy to digest, making it an excellent food during times of digestive discomfort, which can sometimes accompany smoking cessation. It can be made into a gruel (a thin porridge). Slippery elm works with the body to draw out impurities and toxins, assisting with the healing of the entire body. Slippery elm's coating action also soothes the irritated tissues of the intestines, colon, and stomach ulcers, making it a most useful herb for the digestive issues that may accompany smoking cessation. Slippery elm has no known warnings or contraindications.

**Valerian** *(Valeriana officinalis):* Valerian root is one of the premier sedative herbs used to aid people with anxiety, stress, and insomnia. Valerian also acts as a muscle relaxant. Valerian has been commonly used for insomnia and nervous conditions for many centuries. It was a very popular sleep sedative in the United States until the advent of pharmaceutical drugs in the post–World War II era. Clinical studies have shown that valerian root significantly improves sleep quality without morning grogginess. Some researchers have compared valerian root to drugs such as Valium. Valerian, however, is a much milder, safer sedative and is not addictive, nor does it promote dependency. Valerian is clearly one of the herbs of choice in smoking cessation to deal with the issues of insomnia, restlessness, and anxiety. Valerian is not recommended during pregnancy, or if you suffer from low blood pressure or hypoglycemia.

A formula made by combining liquid extracts of oat seed (50 percent), licorice root (25 percent), and lobelia (25 percent) is reported to be particularly useful in overcoming tobacco addiction. Licorice root is included to help with cleansing the lungs and promoting adrenal gland function.

## Hypnosis

This is a technique that has been used successfully by many smokers to kick the habit. Smoking is an addiction, both physiological and psychological. Research tells us that our bodies eliminate the majority of nicotine within a few days after smoking is stopped, essentially rectifying the physiological component of the addiction. But it is the psychological component that continues to drive the desire to smoke. As mentioned before, smoking cigarettes has attached itself to every aspect of your life. In order to defeat the psychological component, there are many behaviors and associations that must be unlearned and replaced by healthy behaviors and associations.

Hypnosis is an excellent tool for this process. Through hypnosis sessions, the therapist will help you change your subconscious motivations to smoke, and in so doing you will change the habits and associations that drive the psychological component of your smoking behavior. Be sure to find a hypnotherapist who has experience helping people quit smoking. Appendix 1 contains information that can help you find a qualified hypnotherapist.

## Nicotine Patches and Nicotine Gum

Nicotine replacement therapy utilizes various forms of nicotine delivery methods that are intended to replace the nicotine that was obtained from smoking or other forms of tobacco usage without the devastating consequences to the lungs and the body that are caused by those habits. These products help with smoking-cessation efforts by reducing withdrawal symptoms and cravings caused by the loss of nicotine from cigarettes. Nicotine replacement therapy allows individuals to wean themselves off nicotine more gradually.

The most common forms of nicotine replacement therapy are nicotine patches and nicotine gum. Nicotine replacement therapy is considered to be useful and beneficial for smokers who are earnestly committed to quitting. With the nonprescription availability of nicotine patches and gum, these two aids for smoking cessation have risen in popularity. Bear in mind that although nicotine patches and gum can help alleviate physical cravings for nicotine, quitting will still require a great amount of effort and willpower.

### Experimental Nicotine Vaccine

Although it is not yet available for the public, Swiss researchers reported in May 2005 that an experimental vaccine against nicotine helped smokers to stop smoking. In a study involving 341 heavy smokers, 42 percent of them were able to quit (continuously abstain from nicotine) for twelve months after receiving the vaccine. Much more testing is required, but the manufacturer (Zurich-based Cytos Biotechnology) hopes to have the vaccine on the market by 2010.

### Smoking-Cessation Programs and Support Groups

A variety of programs are available to help people quit smoking. Below is a small sampling of the kinds of programs and resources you can choose from. I encourage you to explore the many options and approaches to quitting, then select the one that matches your needs and preferences.

#### NICOTINE SOLUTIONS

This smoking-cessation program, in existence since 1978, claims to have helped thousands of individuals to learn how to permanently kick the habit. The Nicotine Solutions program is designed to end your smoking addiction gradually by allowing you to still smoke as you begin the program. The program is predicated on the idea that there is no need to go cold turkey or to deal with withdrawal symptoms when you finally quit. Instead, you learn how to *let your habit die of neglect*. The eight-week-long program walks you through the process of quitting step-by-step, with a multifaceted approach that teaches you how to detoxify, deal with stress and emotions without a cigarette, and regulate your blood sugar level. You learn how to substitute a breathing technique for smoking to get the same "head rush" a cigarette provides. The program also gives you the tools you need to help you avoid gaining weight. One full year of follow-up and group support from your instructor as well as former graduates is included to help make sure you succeed over the long haul.

Nicotine Solutions is located at 2394 Mariner Square Drive #124, Alameda, CA 94501-1023. It can be reached at (866) 735-3580 or on the Web at www.nicotinesolutions.com.

## NICOTINE ANONYMOUS

Nicotine Anonymous is a nonprofit organization that uses an adapted version of the twelve-step Alcoholics Anonymous (AA) program to help committed individuals achieve abstinence from nicotine in any form. Group support and recovery are core components of this program. Like AA, it offers group meetings where people help each other to live nicotine-free lives. Nicotine Anonymous welcomes anyone who is seeking freedom from nicotine addiction, including people who are using other smoking-cessation programs and nicotine withdrawal methods. For more information or to find a meeting near you, call (415) 750-0328 or go to its Web site: www.nicotine-anonymous.org.

## PALO ALTO MEDICAL FOUNDATION

At various locations throughout northern California, the Palo Alto Medical Foundation offers an eight-session group program that utilizes a positive behavior change approach to smoking cessation. People in the group will learn how to develop a quitting strategy, how to deal with recovery symptoms, how to manage stress through relaxation, how to control weight, and also how to develop assertiveness techniques. These programs are offered in partnership with the American Lung Association and various county health departments. For more information, call (408) 523-3222.

## AMERICAN LUNG ASSOCIATION

The American Lung Association offers a free online smoking cessation program that consists of seven modules that guide you through the process of quitting smoking. Go to www.lungusa.org and click the Freedom From Smoking link to preview the program.

## THE GREAT AMERICAN SMOKEOUT

Every year on the third Thursday in November, the American Cancer Society sponsors the Great American Smokeout. On this day, smokers are challenged to quit at least for that day with the hope that it will initiate a lifelong commitment to quitting. In many communities, local volunteers publicize the event and support smokers in their quest to quit. For more information about the Great American Smokeout or about support for quitting in your area, call (800) ACS-2345.

## HOSPITAL-BASED PROGRAMS

Most hospitals regularly sponsor smoking-cessation programs. The types of programs will vary from one facility to another. Contact your local hospital for information on what it offers.

If you are unable to attend program meetings or prefer to participate in online programs or support groups, I recommend visiting the following Web sites:

www.whyquit.com/freedom.html
www.quitsmoking.about.com/mpboards.htm
www.quitsmokingsupport.com/
www.smoking-cessation.org/

### *A Note about Homeopathy*

There is no specific homeopathic remedy for smoking cessation, but a skilled homeopathic practitioner can be very helpful in selecting a remedy that will be useful in helping you achieve your overall comprehensive healing goals, of which smoking cessation is a part. Refer to the section on homeopathy in chapter 7 for a review of the basic principles of homeopathic therapeutics. Appendix 1 contains information to find a qualified homeopathic practitioner.

In addition to the cessation methods just discussed, which are specifically aimed at assisting you in controlling the physical craving for cigarettes, many other techniques can help break the psychological addiction. Yoga, for example, which is discussed elsewhere in this book as a method for addressing the breathing issues related to COPD, is also very useful as a tool in smoking cessation because it helps you to retrain your breathing process as well as relax. An exercise program in general is extremely useful because it improves your fitness, which makes you look and feel better and changes your psychological focus from the deterioration of health to building health. Something as simple as increasing your water intake, which is also discussed elsewhere in this book as an important means to help with the mucus secretions related to COPD, will also help your body cleanse itself of the toxins you have acquired through smoking. Positive affirmations and continual positive self-reinforcement (always reminding yourself of your goals) will enable you to stay mentally focused and engaged in your attempts to quit. In order to succeed, you need to be very proactively involved, self-aware, and focused on what you are trying to achieve—becoming a nonsmoker for life.

## WHAT TO EXPECT WHEN YOU QUIT

When you are about to take on a difficult task, knowing what you are up against can help you prepare and gather your strength for the obstacles you will be facing. The following are complaints and symptoms that are experienced by smokers as they undergo the initial phases of smoking cessation. Some of these problems are related to the physical addiction and some to the psychological addiction. These problems and feelings may be particularly strong for the first days or weeks, but they will ease with time. For each of the problems listed, I have included suggestions about how to combat them and maintain your resolve to be a nonsmoker.

1. **Craving a cigarette:** This is caused by withdrawal from nicotine. When this happens, wait out the urge, as it will last only for a few minutes. Go for a walk around the block or do some other type of exercise. Try the three D's—*distract* yourself, practice *deep breathing,* and *drink water.*

2. **Restlessness/irritability:** This results from your body craving nicotine. When this happens, take a quick walk and/or take a hot bath or shower, and practice relaxation techniques (deep breathing, meditation, and yoga, for example).

3. **Decreased ability to focus or concentrate:** This is happening because your body needs time to adjust from not being constantly stimulated by nicotine. If possible, lighten your workload. Take things a little easier and avoid stress—at least for the first couple of weeks after you quit.

4. **Trouble sleeping:** Not being able to sleep as well at night is due to the fact that nicotine affects brain wave function and sleep patterns. Until this resolves itself, avoid any caffeine after 6 p.m. and perform relaxation techniques before going to bed.

5. **Fatigue:** You're likely to feel tired more often because your body is used to running on a stimulant that you are no longer supplying. Take naps, and until your body chemistry reestablishes itself, don't push yourself as much.

6. **Headache:** This is occurring in all likelihood because your brain is being deprived of nicotine, which it is used to having. It is a common withdrawal symptom. You may resolve this by doing deep breathing exercises, taking a warm bath or shower, using

cool compresses on your forehead, or taking the herb white willow bark (follow instructions on the label).

7. **Hunger:** This is often misconstrued as a craving for a cigarette and it is also related to the oral craving associated with smoking. As this may occur frequently for some, drink either water or another type of low-calorie drink, and satisfy the pangs with low-calorie snacks.

8. **Abdominal pain, gas, constipation:** The movement of your bowels will slow down for a brief time after you quit smoking because your intestines are used to being stimulated by nicotine. Drink plenty of fluids and increase the amount of fiber in your diet by eating more fruits and vegetables and whole grains.

9. **Dizziness:** This is probably due to the fact that your body is now getting more oxygen than it is used to. Your body actually needs to adjust to receiving the amount of oxygen it was meant to have. Be cautious in your movement and change positions slowly.

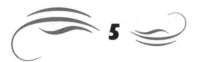

# Dietary Therapeutics

To make the most of natural health options for COPD, you will most likely need to make some significant changes in your diet. After quitting smoking, dietary considerations are by far the most important element of natural healing for your COPD. If you don't change your diet, all the other steps you take to help yourself will be much less effective. Dietary change is the foundation of an overall therapeutic approach whose aim is to build health and lessen the exacerbations that are often seen in COPD.

The advantage of nutrition and other natural therapies over conventional treatments is that they aim not just to address symptoms, but also to reduce inflammation, heal damaged tissue, restore biochemical balance, and otherwise correct problems at a fundamental level. There is no treatment yet that can completely restore the interalveolar septa or the alveoli that have been destroyed in emphysema. There is also no method to restore bronchial walls that have become permanently dilated because of bronchiectasis. However, nutritional and other natural therapies offer many ways to reduce further destruction and to strengthen the remaining lung tissue that has not yet been damaged.

What is implied by the use of the word *diet* as it pertains to COPD is a complete and permanent change in the way you eat for the rest of your life. Permanently changing the way you eat may prove to be one of the most difficult things you must do. However, as you begin to see how much it helps lessen the severity of your COPD symptoms, you will come to welcome your dietary changes as a means of improving your quality of life.

People with COPD burn many calories in breathing. The dietary protocols outlined here will enable you to obtain all the calories you need. Because individuals with chronic lung disease sometimes find it more difficult to breathe while chewing, you may find it more beneficial to eat five or six slightly smaller meals rather than the standard three meals a day. Smaller meals with less chewing, eaten more frequently, may make it easier for you to eat enough to obtain the calories you need and avoid the breathlessness that can be associated with eating big meals.

## THE ROLE OF NUTRITION IN HEALTH AND HEALING

Scientific research in the field of nutritional biochemistry continues to reveal new information regarding the role of nutrients in human metabolism. Today we not only have a better understanding of the relationship between nutrition and health, but we also understand more about how nutritional therapies can help prevent and eradicate illness.

We all know that we are supposed to "eat right" in order to be healthy, but few Americans have been taught what it means to eat a truly healthful diet. The consequences of poor eating habits are all around us. Heart disease, obesity, cancer, and type 2 diabetes are just some of the health problems that are directly related to the typical American diet.

COPD is not caused by a poor diet, but the severity of its symptoms is definitely influenced by the kinds of foods we eat. The typical American diet of fast food and packaged supermarket food is high in fat, low in fiber, full of dangerous chemicals, and lacking in any appreciable amounts of plant substances. Research shows that eating this way can contribute to inflammation and other health consequences that can lead to the development of chronic diseases. It is sure to exacerbate the serious problem with inflammation that people with COPD already have.

Many of the foods we prefer to eat are full of substances that significantly contribute to inflammation and increase the body's toxicity, which weakens the immune system and increases the stress and demands placed on the liver and kidneys. Many of them are also very high in saturated fats and low in fiber, a combination that also significantly increases your risks for cardiovascular disease. And because the "typical American diet" doesn't really include any appreciable amounts of fresh vegetables and fruits, it denies the body the vital nutrients it needs for proper metabolism, for tissue repair and rebuilding, and for fortifying its defense mechanisms. Feeding your body with fresh whole foods instead can have a significant impact on your COPD symptoms as well as your overall health.

The reality is that the things that we eat on a regular basis—the hamburgers, the pizza, the fried foods, the microwavable foods, the processed foods out of the box or can, the sugary drinks—are things we

## A Word about Orthomolecular Medicine

Orthomolecular physicians practice medicine based on the concept of biochemical individuality. They believe that the amounts of nutrients needed to maintain optimal health vary according to each individual's unique biochemical needs. You may be most familiar with a concept of nutrition based on the four food groups, the food pyramid, or the U.S. recommended daily allowance (RDA) for vitamins and minerals. Although the U.S. RDA may be adequate to prevent many deficiency diseases, science shows us that the nutritional requirements for any one individual are actually unique and specific to that individual.

Orthomolecular medicine uses a wide range of diagnostic tests to access personal nutritional status. Through these tests, orthomolecular physicians are able to assess an individual's specific nutritional needs. These tests can also reveal nutritional deficiencies that could lead to future health problems. See appendix 2 for ways to learn more about orthomolecular medicine.

should eat only once in a while. This chapter will provide information on how to eat correctly, not only to help you combat the issues of COPD but also to provide maximum benefit for healthful living.

## HOW CHANGING YOUR DIET CAN HELP

By changing the way you eat, you will not only address your COPD symptoms, you will also support your body in the restoration of your overall health. The nutritional protocols explained here work together to help your body heal itself. Even though some of the dietary changes are aimed at helping to reduce specific symptoms, the main goal is to help your body halt or even reverse the processes that have led to the symptoms by rebuilding and restoring your overall health.

Reducing inflammation, decreasing mucus production, and preventing infection are areas in which nutritional therapies can help people with COPD. Because inflammation is central to many of the problems associated with COPD, successfully addressing the underlying problem of chronic inflammation will make it much easier to lessen or eliminate many of the other problems that are associated with COPD.

## THE IMPORTANCE OF DETOXIFICATION

In order for dietary therapies, nutritional supplements, and herbal medicine to have maximal effects on the body, they need a clean, nontoxic environment in which to work. The process of detoxification helps the body rid itself of toxins and residues that may be impairing optimal function of organs, tissues, and cells.

Detoxification is accomplished through two methods. The first is aimed at cleansing the bowel in order to ensure that conditions in the colon are optimal for its proper and efficient function. The second involves helping the liver—the body's main organ of detoxification—rid the body of accumulated toxins. (Chlorophyll and chlorophyllin are dietary supplements that can help support the detoxification process. See chapter 6 for more information on these supplements.)

## Bowel Cleansing

Cleansing the bowel involves removing impacted waste to prevent systemic problems that can result from their buildup. This kind of detox is accomplished mainly by the use of special enemas that irrigate the colon, as well as by maintaining sufficient amounts of fiber in the diet and/or taking fiber supplements such as psyllium. The movement of dietary fiber through the colon helps prevent waste from collecting there.

Inadequate digestion results in undigested residue lingering in the bowel, which will interfere with the proper absorption of the nutrients you are ingesting to help with your COPD. It is therefore important to detoxify your digestive system and your bowel in order to ensure that you obtain maximum absorption and effectiveness of the nutritional protocols you are employing. To this end, it is important to ensure that you have sufficient amounts of fiber in your diet. In addition to increasing your consumption of high-fiber foods, psyllium is one of the best fiber supplements available to ensure regularity of the bowel. Dietary fiber is found only in plant foods: fruits, vegetables, nuts, and grains. Especially good sources of dietary fiber are lentils, black beans, lima beans, peas, artichokes, brussels sprouts, pears, dried figs, apples, blueberries, bran flakes, and oatmeal.

Incorporating raw foods and juices into your daily diet, as described in this chapter, will itself contribute immensely to the detoxification of your digestive system and entire body. It may also be beneficial for you to initiate the cleansing of your bowel by having a colonic irrigation procedure done by a licensed health care provider or colonic hydrotherapist. This is essentially a high-tech enema that has to be done in the office, and it is very effective at cleansing the bowel of toxic debris. If this is not possible for you, as a second choice I recommend enemas on a weekly basis.

## Supporting the Liver

The other method of detoxification is meant to assist the body, and the liver in particular, in ridding itself of toxic buildup that has occurred within the tissues. This toxic buildup occurs as a result of ingesting harmful chemicals in our food, inhaling cigarette smoke and other pollutants, drinking beverages that contain harmful chemicals, and taking drugs, whether recreational or prescription. These substances are all seen as toxins by your liver.

The liver, part of the digestive system, is the body's main organ of detoxification. The liver metabolizes (breaks down) toxins so that they can be eliminated. Toxins from the food we eat, the water we drink, and the air we breathe are all metabolized and broken down by the liver. Tobacco smoke, prescription drugs, and over-the-counter medicines must all be processed by the liver before they can be eliminated from the body.

After the body breaks down toxins in the liver, it eliminates waste through the intestines (in feces), kidneys (urine), and, to a lesser degree, the lungs (breath) and skin (sweat). Cigarettes, other toxins, and a nutrient-poor diet are all sources of stress for the liver and other organs. If the liver is stressed, it may not be able to work properly to detoxify the body. Furthermore, if the intestines are not working correctly, you will have problems with the absorption of nutrients, which will provoke additional problems.

Water is critical to the detoxification process. It is an essential ingredient needed by your liver for its role in the detoxification process and is also needed in order to flush out your system. Water both acts as a solvent for the myriad chemicals that need to be processed and eliminated and is the major constituent of the transport medium through which many toxins are eliminated from the body—mainly the urine. The liver is the workhorse in the detox process. It is in the liver that chemical reactions occur so as to solubilize the waste products of metabolism as well as other toxins. Without water, none of this can occur. Thus in order for the detoxification process to function efficiently, you need a liver that is functioning optimally and you need plenty of water.

If you have been diagnosed with COPD, there is no doubt that you must give your liver some attention and extra support. To help your liver operate efficiently, it is a good idea to supplement with lipotropic factors and milk thistle seed. See chapter 6 for more information on these dietary supplements.

## Fasting

Fasting is often part of the detoxification process; however, I urge the use of extreme caution in fasting for people with emphysema or other forms of COPD. Depending upon your condition, it is entirely possible that your health is too fragile for you to fast safely. If you do want to incorporate fasting as part of a detoxification protocol, do so only at the advice of and under the direct supervision of your physician.

I usually recommend a ten-day combined juice and water fast. For the first three days, the person drinks nothing but pure distilled water. Then we introduce a seven-day juice fast with only fresh juices (although the person should continue to drink water during this time). The person may also take milk thistle herb and lipotropic factors to support the liver. Then we begin to slowly reintroduce whole foods—fresh fruits and raw or slightly cooked vegetables. Then we move on to more hearty foods that are appropriate to the particulars of the individual in question.

By eliminating everything except water, fresh juice, and liver-support herbs for ten days, the body gets a break and a chance to catch up on cycling out all the junk you most likely have been putting into it. In the event you cannot fast, and depending on your particular needs, there are various types of detoxifcation diets that can be used. Consult your health care practitioner.

## THE MEDICINAL USE OF FOOD FOR COPD

This is where the rubber meets the road. You may find changing the way you eat more difficult than taking medications or even herbs and other dietary supplements. However, making the necessary changes to your diet is essential if you want to improve your health on a fundamental level.

You may need to take your time in adjusting to this new way of eating. However, it's important to remember that the more closely you can adhere to the dietary strategies presented here, the better your results will be. If you are faithful in consistently complying with the guidelines outlined—and consistent compliance means daily compliance for the rest of your life—you will find your problems with COPD much easier to manage.

## FOODS TO AVOID

Certain foods promote inflammation and mucus production. Avoiding these foods can help relieve these problems and ease bronchoconstriction for people with COPD. Reducing mucus and inflammation will result in increased breathing capacity as well as a lowered susceptibility to infection. These are all central issues associated with COPD that can be effectively addressed if you are consistent with the following dietary restrictions.

### Animal Foods to Avoid

Red meat and dairy products are known mucus-forming foods. By eliminating them from your diet, you will reduce mucus production not only in your lungs, but also in your intestines, sinuses, and nasal cavity. However, perhaps the most dramatic result of eliminating these animal foods from your diet is the anti-inflammatory effect you will see. Simply eliminating these foods will have effects similar to those of the steroid drugs you may be familiar with, without the side effects these drugs so often cause. This is because these animal foods are the main dietary source of arachidonic acid, which the body can use to produce pro-inflammatory chemicals such as series-4 leukotrienes and series-2 prostaglandins.

People with COPD should avoid red meat, liver, brain, chicken skin, shellfish, egg yolks, and all dairy products, especially milk, cheese, butter, and any other foods containing butterfat. The elimination of these animal foods from the diet plays a significant role in reducing mucus, inflammation, and bronchoconstriction. If you stop eating these foods, you will have effectively eliminated sources of arachidonic acid from your diet. Your body will still be able to manufacture arachidonic acid from linoleic acid on an as-needed basis. However, in terms of the overall picture, if you eliminate your dietary intake of these animal foods, which are the body's main source of arachidonic acid, you will produce considerably less leukotriene B₄. As a result, you will decrease the inflammatory response occurring in your bronchial walls.

Infants need arachidonic acid for brain development, and nursing mothers provide infants with arachidonic acid through breast milk. Nursing mothers do not have to consume animal products in order to produce the arachidonic acid the baby needs as long as they eat enough plant sources of linoleic acid. For other people, there are no negative consequences to eliminating these particular animal foods from the diet.

### White Flour and Other Gluten-containing Products

White flour products include white bread, pasta, and many cereals. The issue here again is mucus production. White flour products are bad food choices to begin with. The processing and chemical bleaching they undergo strips them of nutrients and leaves toxic residues. White flour contains alloxan (a chemical additive used in processing), which studies have shown destroys the beta cells of the pancreas, thereby significantly contributing to diabetes. Alloxan is also toxic to the liver and kidneys. In addition, because wheat is mucus-forming in general due to the gluten it contains, it is an even worse choice for a COPD patient.

Read food labels very carefully, as many processed food products contain gluten in additives or fillers. For example, millers often add wheat flour to non-wheat flours, such as oats. Good, safe alternative choices to gluten-containing foods include nuts, seeds, non-wheat whole grains, and products made from amaranth, millet, corn, brown rice, and quinoa flours. Pastas made from flour derived from amaranth, brown rice, or quinoa are all excellent alternatives to regular white flour pasta made from semolina and pasta made from whole-wheat flour.

### Salt

Excess sodium (salt) in the bloodstream not only can raise blood pressure, it also reduces the amount of water in the tissues of the bronchi and bronchioles, causing the mucus in the respiratory tract to become thicker and more viscous. Increased sodium concentration in your blood results in water being drawn from the tissues into the blood to lower the concentration of salt. Excessive salt also promotes elevation of histamine levels, which further provokes the inflammatory process.

### Fried Foods

Avoid all greasy, fried foods—especially those that have been deep-fried or fried in oils that are high in trans fats. Fried foods are unhealthy for myriad reasons, but they are also mucus-forming and contribute to the inflammation in your bronchial wall. Some examples of fried foods to avoid are French fries and batter-coated fried chicken. A better alternative is organic skinless chicken breast lightly sautéed in garlic and olive oil with some herbs, spices, and lemon.

### Processed Foods and Refined Sugar

Processed foods and junk foods (much of what is to be found in a box or can in the typical grocery store) are very detrimental to health. Processed foods lose valuable nutrients in the manufacturing process, and both processed foods and junk foods are full of additives and artificial ingredients, all of which are toxic to your body and contribute to inflammation, formation of mucus, and the weakening of your immune system. Foods high in salt and refined sugar, including candy, soda pop, and snack foods, although tasty, will aggravate symptoms of COPD. It is important to read labels very carefully and avoid refined sugar and artificial ingredients. Avoid also all the artificial sweeteners that are available today. If you need a sweetener, use honey sparingly.

The bottom line is that I am advocating a fresh, whole foods diet—meaning you should eat foods as close to their natural, unprocessed state as possible. In general, the more processed the food, the less nutritious it will be. Foods in their natural, unprocessed state contain the highest levels of vitamins, minerals, and nutrients and do not contain additives that may be harmful to your health. Ideally this will mean that you go to the market daily or several times a week to obtain fresh fruits, vegetables, poultry, and fish.

*Beverages to Avoid*

Coffee, black tea, and alcohol are all very dehydrating and therefore deleterious to your health. Caffeine contained in coffee, however, is an effective bronchodilator, and thus can be used to relax the bronchial passages and facilitate easier breathing. The use of caffeine for this purpose should be limited to when absolutely necessary to ease breathing during a situation of acute breathlessness, when nothing else is available to help you.

*Gas-forming Foods*

Excess gas can cause abdominal distention (bloating) that can make breathing more difficult for people with COPD. Gas-promoting foods include cabbage, legumes (peas, lentils, peanuts, beans, and other plant foods that are found in pods), broccoli, onions, brussels sprouts, green peppers, radishes, cauliflower, turnips, corn, soybeans, cucumbers, pickles, sauerkraut, apples, apple juice, bananas, melons, prunes, raisins, and avocados. Which foods cause gas is largely an individual matter. What causes gas for one person may not cause gas for another, so pay attention to your body and learn what foods are gas-producing for you.

## FOODS TO EAT REGULARLY

To support your body's efforts to heal itself, your best choices are whole, unprocessed foods (foods in a state as close to natural as possible), especially fresh vegetables and fruits, raw foods (including vegetables and fruits, nuts, and seeds), fresh raw vegetable and fruit juices, cold-water fish, and unrefined gluten-free grains. Regular consumption of raw foods, including fresh raw vegetable and fruit juices, can make a significant contribution to improving your COPD symptoms as well as your overall health.

Always be sure, within the vast variety of healthful choices you have, that you include plenty of dark green leafy vegetables and purple/red varieties of vegetables; beets, radishes, and red onions; blue, purple, and dark red berries; pineapples and papayas. Some purple and red fruits, such as blueberries, raspberries, and red grapes, are high in beneficial antioxidant plant compounds (see chapter 6 for more information). Papaya and pineapple contain helpful digestive enzymes with anti-inflammatory properties, and dark leafy greens are extremely high in vitamins and minerals. Remember to maintain adequate calcium intake in light of your abstinence from dairy products. Excellent plant-based sources of dietary calcium are dark green leafy vegetables, asparagus, broccoli, kale, soybeans, tofu, and watercress. (You may consider taking supplemental calcium if needed.)

Keep in mind that sweet fruits tend to be mucus-forming, so limit the amount of sweet fruit you consume. Sweet fruits are fruits like dates, bananas, dried fruit, figs, and persimmon. Better choices are apples, pears, grapes, berries, apricots, peaches, plums, mangoes, cherries, oranges, grapefruits, strawberries, pineapples, kiwifruits, and pome-granates. It is also important to use only cold-pressed olive oil, flaxseed oil, and hempseed oil in your food. Any of these oils can be added to salads, but use only olive oil for cooking.

I recommend that you eat organic foods as much as possible. Organic food is produced according to standards that require it to be grown without the use of conventional pesticides or fertilizers and not contain genetically modified organisms (GMOs). Organic meat must be produced without the use of antibiotics or growth hormones.

## RAW FOODS

Ideally, as a COPD patient who wants to make significant improvements in your health, your diet should consist of at least 50 percent raw organic food. A raw foods diet means eating foods (plant foods) in their natural, uncooked state. If you have severe inflammation associated with chronic bronchitis, I recommend increasing the amount of raw food in your diet to 75 percent.

The concept of eating a raw foods diet will in all likelihood seem very strange to you at first. However, a raw foods diet is one of the best possible sources of good nutrition available. Despite the absence of animal products, you can obtain the necessary amount of protein in a raw foods diet once you know what you are doing. Switching to a predominantly raw foods diet has helped many seriously ill people to improve their health. Making raw foods a substantial part of your diet will help your body detoxify itself and build immunity, significantly reduce inflammation, and decrease mucus formation, allowing you to breathe easier, regain energy and strength, and foster a new level of vitality and mental acuity.

Raw foods also contain enzymes that help your body more efficiently digest food. More specifically, they contain the enzymes necessary for the digestion of the foods themselves—enzymes that are lost in cooking, which makes it more difficult to digest what we eat. For example, red pepper contains the enzymes needed to digest red pepper—when it is eaten raw. When we cook red pepper, we lose some of those enzymes, making the pepper more difficult to digest.

You will have to determine, depending upon your circumstances, the extent to which you are willing or able to adopt this style of eating. I highly recommend, if it is possible, that you give this a serious effort, as the health benefits and the degree of improvement it will bring to your condition are considerable.

Adopting a raw food diet is in many ways a lifestyle change that is fairly dramatic. This style of eating is not something you can just jump into; you may want to ease into it gradually.

You will need guidance to help you learn how to eat this way. There are many sources of information and books on how to successfully incorporate raw foods and juices into your life (see appendix 2 for some suggestions). The staff at your local health food store, grocery, or farmer's market are also a great source of information. Recipes are available that can enable you to make a raw food version of almost anything you may crave from your old style of eating. Raw food preparation and variety has actually become something of an art form, just like conventional cuisine. Salads, fresh vegetables, avocado, nut milks, tomatoes, wheatgrass juice, raisins and other dried fruits, seaweed, fresh fruits of all types, pumpkin and sunflower seeds, fresh-squeezed citrus juices, vegetable juices, almonds, sprouts, dried apricots, berries—these are but a few of the hundreds and hundreds of food choices you will have within the world of raw foods eating. Some of them may take some getting used to, but don't be afraid to try something new. Experiment and have fun. Through continued exploration of raw foods and juicing, you will come to develop strategies that work best for the specifics of your case.

## JUICING

Fresh, raw fruit and vegetable juices deliver high-quality, concentrated nutrients to your body that are usually assimilated within 30 minutes. Juicing raw vegetables and fruits is particularly beneficial for people with COPD. In order to obtain maximum nutritional benefit from juicing, it is important for you to prepare fresh juice yourself rather than buy it from a store. Commercial juice is usually pasteurized, a process that uses heat to destroy microorganisms and prolong the product's shelf life. The heat of the pasteurization process also destroys many of the nutrients in the juice. Even some of the highest-quality commercial juice products that utilize "flash pasteurization" still lose valuable nutrients in this process. By using your own juicer, you assure yourself that the juice you prepare is pure, tasty, free of any additives or preservatives, and complete with all the nutritional value that nature intended.

Juicing, in similar fashion to raw foods, can significantly aid in the improvement of your overall health status. For someone with COPD, juicing is an excellent means to reduce inflammation and mucus, detoxify the body, and build immunity in order to increase vitality and resistance to infection. The fresh juices of the following fruits and vegetables are particularly useful for people with COPD:

| | |
|---|---|
| Beet root | Grape |
| Broccoli | Leafy greens (especially spinach and kale) |
| Carrot | Radish |
| Celery | Watercress |
| Cucumber | Wheatgrass |

Depending upon the severity of your COPD, I recommend drinking from two to four 8-ounce glasses of fresh juice daily. If your inflammation and mucus are light to moderate, and you are currently not experiencing any exacerbation of your condition, two 8-ounce glasses a day will suffice. If your inflammation and mucus are severe, try drinking four 8-ounce glasses of juice a day until your condition resolves, and after that, drink two 8-ounce glasses per day as a daily regimen.

Make sure that you vary your choices of juices from the list and rotate through all of them regularly. Pay particular attention to carrot juice, as this is a rich source of beta-carotene, a precursor (building block) for vitamin A. Adequate vitamin A intake is critical for people with COPD; it helps increase resistance to infection and improve pulmonary function. (See chapter 6 for more information on vitamin A.) When preparing your vegetable juices, you may want to add a small amount of garlic juice. Garlic enhances the therapeutic efficacy of the raw vegetable juice by acting as a catalyst for the vegetable juice. (A catalyst is a substance that enhances or increases the activity of another substance.) Add just a quarter or half a teaspoon of garlic juice per 12-ounce glass of juice. If you put in too much, it may overpower the raw vegetable juice and become unpleasant to drink.

## Getting Started with Juicing

If you don't already have a juicer, you will need to obtain one if you are serious about juicing for health. Appendix 1 includes some information on choosing a juicer. Next, you will need to find a good source of quality organic produce and begin learning how to prepare produce for juicing. Juicing fresh produce is a fun and easy process to learn, but there are some particulars that must be understood. To help you get familiar with the process, I recommend reading any of the following books: *Juicing for Life,* by Cherie Calbom; *The Juiceman's Power of Juicing,* by Jay Kordich; or *The Juicing Bible,* by Pat Crocker. These well-reputed books will give you a tremendous amount of information on all aspects of juicing.

*Green Drinks*

Green drinks should be part of the daily dietary regimen of every COPD patient. Wheatgrass juice is the number one choice for green drinks. Wheatgrass is high in chlorophyll (the green pigment in plants) and is one of the richest sources of vitamins A, B, and C. It is also a source of calcium, iron, magnesium, phosphorus, potassium, sodium, sulfur, cobalt, zinc, and protein. As discussed in more detail in chapter 6, chlorophyll has been shown to inhibit some carcinogens and cleanses and detoxifies the circulatory and digestive systems.

Wheatgrass for juicing can be purchased in health food stores, or you can try growing it yourself. You can also purchase powdered green food supplements to mix with water or juice. Supplemental chlorophyllin is available in capsule or liquid form. For suggestions on choosing green food supplements, see appendix 1.

## GOOD SOURCES OF PROTEIN

Skinless organic chicken or turkey and various kinds of cold-water fish are all acceptable food choices for sources of protein. Other excellent sources of protein are tofu and most of the varieties of beans as well as nuts and seeds. Soymilk, rice milk, and almond milk are great choices to substitute for regular dairy milk.

*Cold-water Fish*

Cold-water fish such as salmon, albacore tuna, rainbow trout, herring, mackerel, whiting, sardines, and pilchards are not only good sources of protein, they are excellent sources of nutrients called omega-3 essential fatty acids. Omega-3 fatty acids are found in the oil of cold-water fish as well as in certain plant oils. This group of nutrients, essential for human health, should be obtained from food sources—they cannot be manufactured by the body in sufficient amounts. I recommend eating at least three 4-ounce servings of cold-water fish per week. You can also get omega-3 benefits from eating flaxseed and hempseed.

## Omega-3 Essential Fatty Acids and Inflammation

There are three major types of omega-3 essential fatty acids that are ingested in foods and used by the body: alpha-linolenic acid (ALA), eicosapentaenoic acid (EPA), and docosahexaenoic acid (DHA). The body converts ALA to EPA and DHA. Extensive research indicates that omega-3 fatty acids reduce inflammation and help prevent certain chronic diseases such as heart disease and arthritis. These essential fatty acids are also highly concentrated in the brain and appear to be particularly important for cognitive and behavioral function. EPA and DHA both inhibit the conversion of arachidonic acid to leukotriene $B_4$ and inhibit the conversion of arachidonic acid to the pro-inflammatory series-2 prostaglandins.

It is important to maintain an appropriate balance of omega-3 and omega-6 (another essential fatty acid) in the diet, as these two substances work together to promote health. In general, omega-3 fatty acids help reduce inflammation and most omega-6 fatty acids tend to promote inflammation. An inappropriate balance of these essential fatty acids contributes to the development of disease, while a proper balance helps maintain and even improve health. A healthy balance of omega-6 to omega-3 should be 1:1, not exceeding 4:1. Currently the ratio of omega-6 to omega-3 in the typical American diet is around 10:1 and some estimate it to be as high as 30:1. Many researchers believe this imbalance is a significant factor in the rising rate of inflammatory disorders in the United States.

One of the main reasons why there is so much excess omega-6 in the American diet is that omega-6 linoleic acid is the primary oil ingredient added to most processed foods. It is found in many commonly used cooking oils, including sunflower, safflower, corn, cottonseed, and soybean oils. Arachidonic acid is also an omega-6 and is found in egg yolk, meats in general (particularly red meat and organ meats), and other animal-based foods.

When you cut down on the amount of fatty foods (particularly foods fried in the above-mentioned vegetable oils) and meat in your diet while at the same time increasing the amount of cold-water fish and other sources of omega-3 fatty acids, the balance of omega-6 to omega-3 fatty acids will naturally improve.

The last enzyme in the sequence of steps that convert linoleic acid to arachidonic acid is known as delta-5 desaturase. However, given a choice, delta-5 desaturase would "prefer" to convert omega-3 essential fatty acids into eicosapentaenoic acid (EPA) rather than convert linoleic acid into arachidonic acid. What this means in a practical sense is that if you increase your intake of omega-3 rich foods (like cold-water fish and flaxseed) at the same time you restrict your intake of arachidonic acid–containing animal foods (like red meat), your body will naturally produce beneficial EPA. This means that you will end up producing more series-3 prostaglandins, which are beneficial, rather than the pro-inflammatory and bronchoconstricting series-4 leukotrienes and pro-inflammatory series-2 prostaglandins. With less inflammation and bronchoconstriction occurring in your bronchial walls, the airway will become less obstructed, mucus production will decrease, and you will ultimately be able to breathe easier.

## OTHER HEALTHY FOODS

As you make food choices for yourself, remember to orchestrate your diet within the context of a predominantly raw foods diet so as to gain the maximum therapeutic benefit for your COPD. Black bean soup made with lots of onions, for example, is an excellent source of quercetin, an anti-inflammatory compound. Non–white flour products made from amaranth, corn flour, brown rice, and quinoa provide good alternatives for breads, muffins, and pasta that you will be able to enjoy without causing mucus formation or aggravating your condition.

## TABLE 5. DIET AND FOOD SUMMARY

### Avoid

Red meat, liver, brain, chicken skin, shellfish, and egg yolks

Fried or greasy foods

Processed foods and junk foods, including margarine

Dairy products, especially milk, cheese, and butterfat

White flour products including bread, pasta, cereals derived from white flour, rye, oats, barley, triticale, and whole wheat

Refined sugar products such as candy, snack foods, and soda pop, as well as artificial sweeteners

Salt

Caffeine and alcohol

Foods you are allergic to

### Good Choices

Cold-water fish such as salmon, albacore tuna, rainbow trout, herring, whiting, mackerel, and sardines

Skinless organic poultry

Hot and spicy foods such as onions, garlic, chilis, mustard, and horseradish

Soy, rice, coconut, and almond milk

Non-wheat flour products, corn flour, brown rice flour, amaranth, and quinoa

Raw foods: all fresh organic fruits and vegetables, nuts, seeds, and non-wheat whole grains

Cold-pressed olive oil, flaxseed oil, hempseed oil

Tofu

Honey, used sparingly

## *Adding Hot and Spicy Foods*

To the extent that your palate can tolerate them, foods such as onions, garlic, various types of chili peppers, mustard, and horseradish will all benefit your condition. These foods are stimulating to your immune system and help provide nourishment to your respiratory system. Furthermore, garlic and onions both contain quercetin, a flavonoid compound that research has shown to inhibit lipoxygenase. Inhibition of lipoxygenase means that the production of series-4 leukotrienes will decrease, which will result in less bronchoconstriction and inflammation. Research also indicates that quercetin can inhibit pro-inflammatory series-2 prostaglandins. Taking supplemental quercetin will further enhance the inhibition of series-4 leukotrienes and the pro-inflammatory series-2 prostaglandins.

By eliminating the animal foods mentioned in this chapter, increasing your intake of foods rich in omega-3 essential fatty acids, and increasing your dietary intake of garlic and onions, you will very effectively inhibit the formation of pro-inflammatory series-2 prostaglandins and series-4 leukotrienes. This will reduce bronchoconstriction, inflammation, and the production of mucus, which will enable you to breathe easier and lower your susceptibility to infection.

## PROPER FOOD COMBINING

When a food is eaten together with other foods, its effect on the body can be significantly altered. To ensure proper digestion and to help reduce mucus formation and inflammation, it is essential to combine foods appropriately.

Figure 7 on page 88 is a guide to proper food combining. Following these guidelines will improve the efficiency of your digestion and minimize inflammation and mucus. You may combine foods from boxes that are directly connected by an arrow, but you should combine foods from only two boxes at a time. Melon should always be eaten alone.

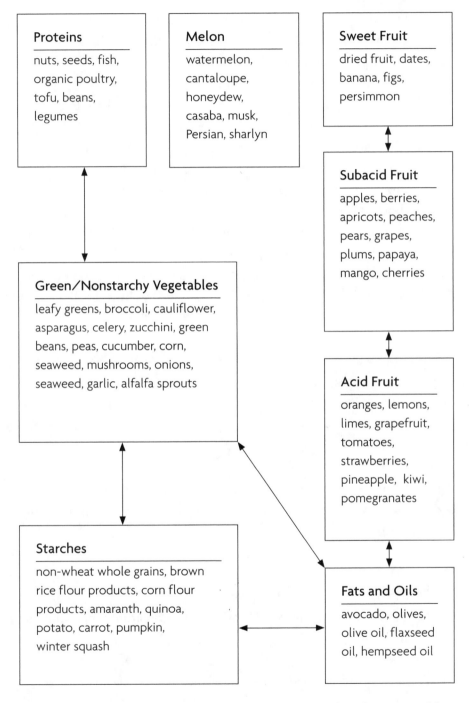

*Fig. 7. Proper Food Combining. Foods in boxes that are directly connected by an arrow may be eaten at the same meal.*

1. Do not eat proteins and starches together. Proteins and starches eaten together tend to spoil in the stomach, cause indigestion and fatigue, and promote weight gain.
2. Do not eat proteins with fats or oils.
3. Eat proteins as a main course with vegetables and a salad.
4. Eat starches as a main course with vegetables and a salad.
5. Always eat fruit by itself on an empty stomach. Allow a half-hour to pass after eating fruit before eating other foods. Melon should be eaten either alone or before other fruits. Sweet fruits should be eaten after other fruits.
6. You may eat nuts with acid fruits (such as citrus fruits, pineapple, strawberries, and pomegranate).
7. Avocados combine well with all foods except proteins and melons.
8. Tomatoes may be combined with non-starchy vegetables and protein.

The following guidelines will show you how to combine food when eating so as to streamline digestion, reduce mucus formation, and energize and strengthen your body.

## HEALTHY MEAL IDEAS

The following lists of foods for each meal of the day are provided to show you how all this information on healthy eating translates into healthy meals.

### BREAKFAST
Fresh vegetable and/or citrus juice
Cereals made from non-wheat grains such as amaranth, rice, quinoa, and millet
Nuts and/or seeds
Fresh fruit and/or dried fruits and/or melon

## LUNCH (CAN ALSO BE DINNER CHOICES)

Vegetable stir-fry with a few cashews or walnuts over a bed of non-wheat grains such as rice, quinoa, and millet

Corn tostada layered with low-fat refried beans with sliced avocado, salsa, and shredded carrots

Non-wheat pasta (made from amaranth, quinoa, millet, or rice) with fresh tomato sauce or fresh garlic and olive oil

Grilled chicken breast (organic and skinless) with fresh, lightly steamed vegetables

Fresh vegetable juices made in your juicer

Fresh salads sprinkled with flaxseed or hempseed

Fresh salad with marinated tofu and Dijon-vinaigrette dressing

Assorted sushi (mainly salmon, halibut, tuna, yellowtail; no shellfish) with wasabi and edamame and seaweed salad

Assorted nuts, fresh fruits

## DINNER (CAN ALSO BE LUNCH CHOICES)

Lightly baked or broiled salmon drizzled with lemon and olive oil served with fresh steamed vegetables

Fajitas with grilled skinless organic chicken on corn tortillas with guacamole, tomatoes, lettuce, and black olives served with rice and black beans

Lightly pan-sautéed rainbow trout with lemon, served with rice pilaf and lightly grilled vegetables

Hearty vegetable soup with a fresh raw salad

## HYDRATION AND THE CRITICAL ROLE OF WATER

One of the simplest yet most effective ways to help with the mucus problem of COPD is to ensure adequate hydration—making sure that you drink sufficient amounts of water. By water, I mean pure water, not iced tea, lemonade, or other beverages made with water. In order for water to be efficiently utilized by your body, it must be consumed in its pure form.

Most people are chronically dehydrated because of inadequate water intake. Digestive problems, compromised organ function, arthritis, bladder problems, obesity, diabetes, arteriosclerosis, kidney stones, and headaches are just a few of the health issues that are either related to or aggravated by inadequate water consumption. Your body is composed of approximately 70 percent water, which makes water one of the most important molecules in your body. If you do not consume enough pure water, many physiological functions become compromised. Proper transport of nutrients throughout your body, blood circulation, efficient excretion of wastes and sweating, maintenance of blood pressure and body temperature, and myriad chemical reactions in the body all depend upon an adequate supply of water.

For people with COPD, proper hydration also helps to reduce the viscosity of their mucus secretions. This will enable you to expectorate mucus with much greater ease and with less physical effort in coughing. This may sound too simple to be true, but it is a proven fact that sufficient hydration helps reduce the viscosity of mucus secretions from the respiratory tract. Despite its simplicity, however, drinking enough water is still difficult for many people to do.

You have probably learned that in order to maintain adequate hydration, you should drink between eight and ten 8-ounce glasses of water a day. That amounts to a total of 64 to 80 ounces of pure water daily. This is a rather arbitrary amount that takes no account of the specifics of your own body. A much more accurate way to calculate the amount of water you should be drinking, especially to help lessen the viscosity of mucus secretions, is based on your body weight. In order to maintain adequate hydration for essential bodily functions, as well as to help reduce mucus viscosity, you should drink between half and two thirds of your body weight in ounces of water per day.

Let me show you how to calculate this for yourself. One half is 50 percent, or .5. Two thirds is 66 percent, or .66. To figure out approximately how much water to drink a day, first multiply your body weight by .5, and then multiply your body weight again by .66. Your answers will represent fractions of your body weight, which will give you a range of how many ounces of water to drink a day. For example, if you weigh 150 pounds, your answers will be 75 and 99. These numbers tell you that if you weigh 150 pounds, you should drink between 75 and 99 ounces of water daily. Table 6 provides more examples of water-per-body-weight calculations.

You can see that the theory of eight to ten 8-ounce glasses a day is only adequate for a person who weighs 125 pounds. For people who weigh less than 125 pounds, this amount would over-hydrate them, which is not healthy either, and for people who weigh more than 125 pounds, this amount leaves them under-hydrated. The heavier you are, the more water you need. *Note:* People who have kidney disease, who are taking diuretics to treat blood pressure, or who have neurological or psychiatric disorders should consult with their physician to make sure it is safe for them to consume the recommended amounts of water.

### TABLE 6. CALCULATING DAILY WATER INTAKE

| Body weight | Multiplied by one half (.5) | Multiplied by two thirds (.66) | Adequate daily water intake* |
|---|---|---|---|
| 100 pounds | 100 x .5 = 50 | 100 x .66 = 66 | 50 to 66 ounces |
| 125 pounds | 125 x .5 = 62.5 | 125 x .66 = 82.5 | 63 to 83 ounces |
| 150 pounds | 150 x .5 = 75 | 150 x .66 = 99 | 75 to 99 ounces |
| 175 pounds | 175 x .5 = 87.5 | 175 x .66 = 115.5 | 88 to 116 ounces |
| 200 pounds | 200 x .5 = 100 | 200 x .66 = 132 | 100 to 132 ounces |
| 225 pounds | 225 x .5 = 112.5 | 225 x .66 = 148.5 | 113 to 149 ounces |
| 250 pounds | 250 x .5 = 125 | 250 x .66 = 165 | 125 to 165 ounces |

*16 ounces = 1 pint; 32 ounces = 1 quart; 64 ounces = 1 half-gallon; 128 ounces = 1 gallon

People who are dehydrated actually tend to retain water because their bodies try to compensate for the lack of water they receive. This contributes to obesity. If you are overweight but give your body the water it requires to carry out its metabolic business, you will find that not only will you not retain water, but you will actually begin to lose weight and start feeling much better as well.

As a final point: the quality of the water you drink is of the utmost importance to your health. It is essential that you drink only pure, clean water, so you may need to purchase bottled water or install a water filter on your tap. I highly recommend that you not drink unfiltered tap water from municipal sources. Depending upon its source and method of treatment, municipal tap water may contain many harmful chemicals, including radon, fluoride, arsenic, iron, lead, copper, fertilizers, asbestos, cyanide, herbicides, pesticides, industrial chemicals, viruses, bacteria, parasites, chlorine, carbon, lime, phosphates, soda ash, and aluminum sulfate.

One good option is to drink water that has been filtered by reverse osmosis. You can obtain bottled water that has been filtered in this manner, or you may purchase a water-filtering unit that attaches to your sink. Commercially available filtering systems that use activated carbon are suitable as well. Bottled springwater can also be an acceptable choice as long as you are able to buy it from a reputable source. If you have a well, periodically have your water tested to be sure there is no contamination of groundwater in your area.

The great physician Hippocrates once said, "Let your food be your medicine and let your medicine be your food." You may feel some apprehension at present because my suggestions about changing your diet appear pretty drastic. Be patient with yourself. It may take several months for you to establish yourself in your new dietary patterns. The point is to work at it every day and see yourself making progress toward improving your condition. Once you begin to see the difference these dietary changes have made in your health, you will be more than glad that you chose to make them.

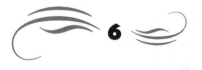

# Dietary Supplements

Dietary supplements can be a valuable part of a complete, holistic program of natural health care for COPD. Supplements are best used in combination with dietary and other lifestyle changes. In other words, if you don't quit smoking and change your diet, dietary supplements probably won't help as much with your COPD. But if used correctly, dietary supplements not only help provide relief from some of the symptoms of COPD, but they also support the body's overall healing process in myriad ways. Dietary supplements include vitamins, minerals, herbal remedies, other plant-based preparations (such as plant oils), enzymes, amino acids, and other natural substances and nutrients.

## USING DIETARY SUPPLEMENTS
## SAFELY AND EFFECTIVELY

You might find that taking dietary supplements is a little easier than making dietary and other lifestyle changes, because you are already accustomed to taking medications for COPD.

Most of the supplements described here should be taken orally in pill or capsule form. Some supplements come in liquid form, and most of these liquid supplements should be either taken orally or inhaled using a nebulizer (a device designed to allow medications to be inhaled directly into the lungs). You may already be familiar with how to use a nebulizer unit because this is probably the way in which you take your albuterol or other bronchodilator medications.

To ensure safety with dietary supplements, always exercise responsibility and care when using them. Learn as much as you can about the effects of supplements, and do not exceed recommended dosages. One of the major benefits of dietary supplements is that they usually cause fewer and less dangerous side effects than pharmaceutical drugs. But some dietary supplements can have side effects if used incorrectly or inappropriately. Many people think that vitamins, herbs, and other dietary supplements are always safe just because they are "natural." This is not true.

With all the information about dietary supplements now available in books, on the Internet, and in the media, it is easy to become confused about what dietary supplements to take. Again, it is extremely important that you work with an experienced health care professional who not only is familiar with your case, but is also trained to be able to advise you about which supplements may benefit you most, and at what dosages. Your health care provider will be able to help you determine which of the supplements discussed here will be most helpful for your particular case.

### A Note about Blood-thinning Substances

Certain dietary supplements are believed to have the potential to cause "blood-thinning" effects. Among others, some blood-thinning drugs and supplements are warfarin (Coumadin); aspirin and other nonsteroidal anti-inflammatory drugs (NSAIDs) such as ibuprofen; fish and plant oils rich in omega-3 fatty acids; enzymes; and certain herbal supplements, including garlic, ginger, and ginkgo. Be cautious about using these drugs or supplements in combination with each other, and always discontinue the use of such substances before surgery. You will find specific information about blood-thinning effects in the safety information provided for supplements discussed here.

## USING A NEBULIZER

A nebulizer unit provides a highly effective way to deliver liquid supplements and medications directly into the respiratory tract. A nebulizer unit consists of a small air compressor (usually smaller than a shoebox) that forces compressed air through a tube into a container (the nebulizer) that holds a small amount of liquid. When the compressed air passes through the nebulizer holding the liquid, it changes the liquid into a mist. This mist passes through the opening on the lid of the nebulizer into a tube that leads to a mouthpiece or a mask. The person using the nebulizer inhales the mist directly into the lungs over a period of about 5 to 20 minutes, depending upon how much liquid is in the nebulizer.

A good-quality home nebulizer unit can be purchased online or through many medical supply stores. They may also be obtained through your physician. Prices range from about $60 to $150. The nebulizer containers, masks or mouthpieces, and tubing must be replaced from time to time at a nominal cost. You can find more information about choosing and purchasing a nebulizer in appendix 1.

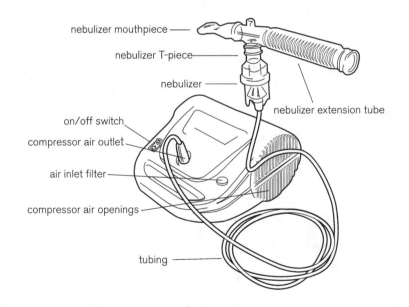

nebulizer mouthpiece

nebulizer T-piece

nebulizer

nebulizer extension tube

on/off switch

compressor air outlet

air inlet filter

compressor air openings

tubing

*Fig. 8. Nebulizer compressor, tubing, nebulizer container, and mouthpiece.*

## DIETARY SUPPLEMENTS AND COPD

In order to understand how dietary supplements can help with COPD, it is necessary to have a general understanding of some of the effects they have upon the body. Some dietary supplements have anti-inflammatory effects, while others help break up mucus. Many dietary supplements provide a number of different actions that complement one another. For example, the enzyme serrapeptase is anti-inflammatory and helps break up mucus.

The information provided here is intended to serve as a starting point for learning about the effects of dietary supplements. The more you learn about dietary supplements on your own, the better able you will be to make informed choices.

---

### Free Radicals, Antioxidants, and Lung Health

An antioxidant is a substance that can protect the cells of the body from the damaging effects of unstable molecules called *free radicals.* Free radicals are found in cigarette smoke, other pollutants, certain unhealthy foods, and many other sources. They have been linked with the development of numerous diseases, including cancer and heart disease. Antioxidants are compounds that can combat the damaging effects of these unstable free radical molecules. Antioxidants are widely found in plant foods, such as fresh fruits and vegetables, and include certain vitamins and various beneficial plant chemicals.

In chemical terms, free radical molecules are unstable because they lack an electron in their outer shell. In order to stabilize themselves, they react with whatever they can to get the electron they need to stabilize their outer shell. For example, when free radicals from cigarette smoke enter into lungs, they "steal" electrons from the molecules that make up lung tissue in an effort to stabilize themselves. This causes what is known as *oxidative damage.* The free radical in the cigarette smoke stole an electron from a molecule

---

that was part of a cell within the lung, leaving that lung cell with a damaged molecule. Over the course of time, as thousands of lung cells are damaged by free radicals, this oxidative damage contributes to the deterioration of lung health.

Free radicals, such as those found in cigarette smoke, can damage the lungs in several ways. Free radicals react with alpha-1 antitrypsin (alpha-1 AT) so that alpha-1 AT cannot do its job of preventing elastase from degrading elastin in the alveolar wall. Free radicals also contribute to inflammation in the lungs, and free radical damage to the surface of lung cells can lead to lung cancer.

*Antioxidants* help combat free radical damage by stabilizing free radical molecules. In very simple terms, an antioxidant molecule can provide the electron missing from the free radical so it doesn't have to steal it from the cell. The antioxidant prevents the free radical from doing oxidative damage by donating an electron to the free radical. This is why it is so important to have a diet rich in fresh fruits and vegetables, including (but not limited to) grapes, raspberries, strawberries, blackberries, cherries, cantaloupe, plums, broccoli, celery, onions, cabbage, and parsley. These natural foods contain abundant amounts of antioxidants, and a diet rich in fresh fruits and vegetables ensures that a wide variety of antioxidants is always available to combat the ongoing threat of oxidative damage.

Antioxidants can help people with COPD in a number of ways. By stabilizing free radicals, antioxidants help lessen inflammation and prevent further destruction of lung tissue. With fewer free radicals present, there is less recruitment of neutrophils to the lungs and thus less inflammation. In addition, alpha-1 antitrypsin is better able to do its job in preventing elastase from destroying elastin.

The following list explains the terms that will be used to describe the particular actions of dietary supplements that are helpful in COPD.

*Anti-inflammatory.* Anti-inflammatory supplements can help reduce underlying inflammation in the respiratory tract. Supplements with anti-inflammatory benefits appear to exert their actions by inhibiting the actions of enzymes that produce pro-inflammatory chemicals in the body.

*Antimicrobial.* Antimicrobial substances kill or render inactive disease-causing organisms (also known as pathogens) that can lead to infection. Antibacterial, antifungal, and antiviral agents are all part of this category.

*Antioxidant.* Antioxidants help the body protect itself against damage from unstable chemical compounds called oxidants, also known as free radicals.

*Bronchodilator.* Substances with bronchodilator actions help relax constricted muscles in the bronchi and bronchioles.

*Immunomodulator.* Immunomodulators have effects on the function of the immune system, the body's built-in system of defense against disease. By boosting the immune system's disease-fighting abilities, immunomodulator supplements may be able to help people with COPD avoid respiratory tract infections.

*Mucolytic.* Mucolytic supplements thin and break up mucus so it can be expectorated (expelled) more easily.

For overall health, daily consumption of a multivitamin and mineral complex is essential for every COPD patient. (For suggestions on choosing a high-quality multivitamin and mineral formula, see appendix 1.) If you are pregnant, nursing, or taking pharmaceutical medications, consult with your health care practitioner before using any dietary supplement. For dosage information, follow manufacturer's recommendations, or consult a health care practitioner familiar with treating COPD.

TABLE 7.

## SUMMARY OF ACTIONS FOR NUTRITIONAL SUPPLEMENTS

| Supplement | Actions* |
| --- | --- |
| Bromelain | Anti-inflammatory, **mucolytic** |
| Chlorophyll/ chlorophyllin | **Detoxification**, cancer preventive |
| Colloidal silver | **Antimicrobial**, anti-infective |
| Dimethylglycine | Antioxidant, **enhances utilization of oxygen by cells**, immunomodulator |
| Evening primrose oil | **Anti-inflammatory** |
| Fish oil | **Anti-inflammatory**, helps lower cholesterol and triglycerides, can help prevent high blood pressure |
| Flaxseed oil | **Anti-inflammatory,** may help prevent heart disease and cancer |
| *Ginkgo biloba* extract | **Anti-inflammatory**, antioxidant, inhibits bronchoconstriction, helps increase blood flow to the tissues and organs |
| Glutathione | **Antioxidant** |
| Grape seed extract | Anti-inflammatory, **antioxidant**, protects heart health |
| Hempseed oil | **Anti-inflammatory** |
| Inosine | **Anti-inflammatory**, antioxidant, immunomodulator |
| Lactoferrin | **Antimicrobial** |
| Lipotropic factors | **Liver support** |
| Magnesium | **Bronchodilator** |
| Manganese | **Anti-inflammatory**, antioxidant |
| Milk thistle extract | Antioxidant, **liver protective** |
| *N*-acetylcysteine (NAC) | Antioxidant, **mucolytic** |

*The most important actions are highlighted in boldface type.

### TABLE 7. ACTIONS FOR NUTRITIONAL SUPPLEMENTS (CONT.)

| Supplement | Actions* |
|---|---|
| Oregano essential oil | **Antimicrobial**, anti-inflammatory, antioxidant, expectorant (mucolytic) |
| Pycnogenol | Anti-inflammatory, **antioxidant** |
| Quercetin | Antioxidant, **anti-inflammatory** |
| Selenium | **Antioxidant** |
| Serrapeptase | **Anti-inflammatory, mucolytic** |
| Superoxide dismutase | **Antioxidant** |
| Vitamin A | **Immunomodulator**, promotes healthy mucous membranes in the respiratory tract, general health benefits |
| Vitamin B complex | **Tissue repair**, general health benefits |
| Vitamin C | Anti-inflammatory, **antioxidant**, immunomodulator, tissue repair, general health benefits |
| Vitamin E | Anti-inflammatory, **antioxidant** |
| Zinc | **Anti-inflammatory**, immunomodulator |

*The most important actions are highlighted in boldface type.

## THE SUPPLEMENTS

### Bromelain

**Main actions:** Anti-inflammatory, mucolytic

Bromelain is the name given to a group of enzymes derived from the pineapple plant. These enzymes (called proteolytic enzymes) are well known to help with digestion, and research shows that they also have anti-inflammatory effects. Bromelain helps decrease the viscosity (thickness) of mucus secretions in chronic bronchitis. The activity of bromelain is enhanced when combined with quercetin and vitamin C.

**Safety information:** Vomiting, diarrhea, cramps, and menstrual problems have occasionally been reported. People using blood-thinning drugs or supplements (anticoagulants or antithrombotic agents) should be cautious with bromelain, as it may enhance the activity of these substances. Bromelain has also been reported to increase blood levels of the antibiotics amoxicillin and tetracycline. Do not use bromelain if you are pregnant or nursing.

**Dosage advice:** Tablets: 500–2,000 GDUs (gelatin digestion units), one to three times daily. Take bromelain on an empty stomach.

## Chlorophyll and Chlorophyllin

**Main action:** Detoxification

Chlorophyll, found in all green plants and available as a dietary supplement, is an important "green food." Chlorophyll is the green pigment in plants. Chlorophyllin is a semisynthetic sodium/copper derivative of chlorophyll. In contrast to chlorophyll, chlorophyllin is water-soluble.

Research indicates that chlorophyll has the ability to protect against several toxins, including certain toxins found in cigarette smoke and coal dust. Experimental data also suggest that chlorophyll and chlorophyllin have antimutagenic and anticarcinogenic potential and may ameliorate some drug side effects. Wheatgrass juice is probably the best natural source of cholorophyll. (See chapter 4 for more information on wheatgrass juice.)

**Safety information:** Discoloration of urine or feces may occur, but this is nothing to worry about.

**Dosage advice:** Follow manufacturer's directions.

## Colloidal Silver

**Main action:** Antimicrobial

Colloidal silver is silver suspended in liquid for oral or inhaled use. Silver has a long history of use as an antimicrobial agent, and the use of colloidal silver as an antimicrobial drug was part of conventional medicine until patented antibiotics were introduced in the 1940s. Colloidal silver may be taken orally or inhaled with a nebulizer (see cautions below).

Silver can kill hundreds of different microorganisms, including methicillin-resistant *Staphylococcus aureus* (MRSA). Researchers believe that colloidal silver works by disabling enzymes that disease-causing organisms are dependent upon. Bacteria do not seem to develop a resistance to silver as they do to antibiotics.

There are many brands of colloidal silver on the market, and they are not all equal. Some of these brands are composed of mainly silver ions or silver protein complexes; these products are not true colloidal silver and should not be used.

**Safety information:** There can be safety concerns with some silver products. Some brands are inappropriately labeled as colloidal silver but are not true colloidal silver; rather, these are products made with a high silver ion content or are silver protein products. These products (ionic silver and silver protein products) may contribute to the development of argyria (an irreversible condition in which the skin turns bluish gray due to exposure to certain forms of silver). True colloidal silver should not cause argyria and has the highest ratio of pure silver colloids to effectively destroy disease-causing microorganisms. (I recommend that you use a colloidal silver product called Mesosilver; see appendix 1 for more information.)

Individuals allergic to silver should avoid using colloidal silver. Always test colloidal silver on the skin. Place a few drops of colloidal silver on the skin and watch for gray patches that may instantly appear on the skin upon colloidal silver application. If gray discoloration occurs, this means you are allergic and should not utilize silver in any form. The skin discoloration is temporary; it is an indication of an extremely uncommon reaction to silver.

When using colloidal silver in a nebulizer, always watch for signs of increased irritability, loss of concentration, and increased emotional instability. If any of these symptoms occur, cut down or temporarily suspend colloidal silver use. These are signs that signal various silver reactions that may occur when high quantities of colloidal silver are used. These initial signs, if experienced, are temporary. Suspending use will give the body time to adjust and prevent any harm to it.

NOTE: Never nebulize colloidal silver unless you are absolutely sure that you are using a pure colloidal silver product. Silver compounds consisting of large amounts of silver salts, proteins, or other chemical agents, especially silver nitrate, can cause instant and potentially terminal silver poisoning under some conditions.

In cases of severe lung infections, employ extreme caution when nebulizing colloidal silver. When the mist reaches the infected tissues in the lungs, the effects of the colloidal silver as an anti-infective can be almost immediate. If the individual is already weak to the point that breathing is laborious, do not nebulize colloidal silver unless a qualified health care practitioner is present.

Dosage advice: During acute respiratory infection, take 5 ml internally and 5 ml via nebulizer every three to four hours until the infection abates.

It can be beneficial to use cayenne along with colloidal silver. Cayenne very effectively loosens mucus in the lungs, including mucus associated with infections. Within only a few minutes of using cayenne orally, mucus will begin to break up and the lungs will begin to clear. Colloidal silver is only effective in areas it can contact directly. Utilizing cayenne to break up mucus exposes more of the surface lining of the lung tissue to the colloidal silver. This greatly increases the infection-fighting properties of colloidal silver when used in the lungs. Mix one teaspoon of high-quality cayenne powder (90,000–150,000 heat units, or HU) in a glass of warm water. Hold a mouthful under the tongue for at least 30 seconds and then swallow. The discomfort caused by taking cayenne this way is temporary, and this is best done when the stomach is not empty. Wait 5 to 10 minutes and then inhale the colloidal silver via the nebulizer.

## Dimethylglycine (DMG)

**Main actions:** Antioxidant, enhances utilization of oxygen by cells, immunomodulator

The primary benefit of dimethylglycine (DMG) in COPD is that it appears to help enhance the way cells utilize oxygen. DMG is an amino acid with a chemical structure resembling that of a water-soluble vitamin. DMG is found in a variety of grains and seeds; it is also produced naturally by the body and functions as an antioxidant. Dimethylglycine has been found to be effective in supporting immune system function and research continues to explore how it may enhance the utilization of oxygen by cells.

**Safety information:** No adverse effects have been reported with recommended doses. However, excessive doses may cause mild nausea that can last for a couple of days.

**Dosage advice:** Take 125–250 mg as a chewable tablet or sublingual tablet (to be placed under the tongue) one to three times daily.

## Evening Primrose Oil

**Main action:** Anti-inflammatory

Evening primrose oil comes from the seeds of the evening primrose plant *(Oenothera biennis)*. Evening primrose oil is a rich source of omega-6 gamma-linolenic acid (GLA) and its precursor, linoleic acid (LA). Research suggests evening primrose oil may help reduce inflammation through the role it plays in the biochemistry of the eicosanoids. GLA is converted to dihomo-gamma-linolenic acid (DGLA), and DGLA can help reduce inflammation by competitively inhibiting the formation of series-4 leukotrienes and series-2 prostaglandins. When DGLA is metabolized to 15-hydroxyl DGLA, it blocks the conversion of arachidonic acid to series-4 leukotrienes, particularly $LTB_4$, thereby effectively reducing inflammation. Furthermore, DGLA is the precursor molecule to prostaglandin $E_1$ ($PGE_1$), which exerts an inhibitory effect on polymorphonuclear leukocytes. PGE₁ also increases intracellular levels of another cellular messenger molecule known as cyclic AMP (cAMP). An increased level of cAMP reduces the release of lysosomal enzymes, reduces leukocyte chemotaxis, and induces the relaxation of bronchial smooth muscle; relaxing bronchial smooth muscle will lessen bronchoconstriction.

Evening primrose is unique because even though it is an omega-6, it goes down a pathway that ultimately leads to anti-inflammatory action. However, in order to get the full anti-inflammatory benefit available through this strategy, and to maintain the needed balance between the omega-6 and omega-3 fatty acids, you should also supplement with an omega-3 fatty acid such as flaxseed oil, which is an excellent source of omega-3 alpha-linolenic acid (ALA).

**Safety information:** There have been some reports of nausea, vomiting, bloating, flatulence, and diarrhea in people taking evening primrose oil. People with a history of seizure disorders, schizophrenia, or hemophilia should avoid evening primrose oil. People using blood-thinning drugs (anticoagulants or antithrombotic agents) or supplements with blood-thinning effects should be cautious with evening primrose oil, as it may enhance the activity of these substances.

**Dosage advice:** 400–3,000 mg daily in divided doses (capsules).

## Fish Oil

**Main action:** Anti-inflammatory

Fish oil is an excellent source of omega-3 essential fatty acids. Fish oil has undergone extensive clinical research that confirms its anti-inflammatory benefits. For people with COPD, regular consumption of fish oil can help reduce inflammation in the airway, decrease mucus production, and enable them to breath easier. Fish oil supplements are made from the body oils of cold-water fish, which include salmon, sardines, and mackerel. As noted already in chapter 4, cold-water fish should be a core component of your daily diet.

Fish oil is a rich source of the important omega-3 fatty acids eicosapentaenoic acid (EPA) and docosahexaenoic acid (DHA), which can help reduce inflammation. Research suggests that EPA and DHA exert anti-inflammatory actions through their ability to inhibit the conversion of arachidonic acid to leukotriene $B_4$ and series-2 prostaglandins.

In addition to reducing inflammation, studies show that fish oil benefits heart health by lowering blood pressure and triglyceride levels, can relieve some of the symptoms of rheumatoid arthritis, and can help with ulcerative colitis and Crohn's disease, among other effects.

**Safety information:** No adverse effects have been reported. People with diabetes or hemophilia should consult with a doctor before taking a fish oil supplement. People using blood-thinning drugs (anticoagulants or antithrombotic agents) or supplements with blood-thinning effects should be cautious with fish oil, as it may enhance the activity of these substances. Always discontinue the use of fish oil prior to surgery.

**Dosage advice:** Soft gels: 3–5 grams total (combined EPA and DHA) daily in divided doses (capsules) with meals. Formulations are often in a ratio of 1.5:1 EPA to DHA. Check the label for the actual amounts of EPA and DHA.

Be sure the fish oil formula you choose contains vitamin E, which helps protect the fish oil against oxidation.

## Flaxseed Oil

**Main action:** Anti-inflammatory

Flaxseed oil is an excellent source of essential fatty acids, as flax is one of the few plants that contain both omega-3 and omega-6 essential fatty acids. Flaxseed oil consists mainly of omega-3 alpha-linolenic acid (ALA) and is a moderate source of omega-6 linoleic acid (LA). In the body, ALA is metabolized to eicosapentaenoic acid (EPA), which is the precursor of the anti-inflammatory series-3 prostaglandins and series-5 leukotrienes. Research suggests ALA may also inhibit the formation of pro-inflammatory series-2 prostaglandins, leukotriene B$_4$, and pro-inflammatory cytokines.

As a limited source of linoleic acid (LA), which can be converted into gamma-linolenic acid (GLA), flaxseed oil can also contribute to reducing inflammation through the anti-inflammatory actions of dihomo-gamma-linolenic acid (DGLA).

**Safety information:** Flaxseed oil has occasionally been reported to cause diarrhea. People with hemophilia and those using blood-thinning drugs (anticoagulants or antithrombotic agents) or supplements with blood-thinning effects should be cautious with flaxseed oil, as it may enhance the activity of these substances.

**Dosage advice:** Take 1,000–6,000 mg daily in divided doses (capsules). If you are using flaxseed oil as part of your diet, lessen the amount you take as a supplement so as to not exceed 6,000 mg daily.

## Ginkgo biloba Extract

**Main actions:** Anti-inflammatory, antioxidant, enhances microcirculation (circulation of blood in tiny capillaries)

*Ginkgo biloba* standardized extract is well known for its ability to enhance peripheral blood circulation (circulation in tiny blood vessels). Ginkgo also has anti-inflammatory effects that make it useful in COPD.

The herb contains a chemical compound called ginkgolide B, which inhibits the effects of platelet-activating factor (PAF). PAF is a very potent molecule that has effects on many leukocyte functions, platelet aggregation (the clumping together of blood platelets), and inflammation. In addition to causing platelets to aggregate and blood vessels to dilate, it also causes bronchoconstriction. At high enough concentrations, PAF causes life-threatening inflammation of the airways. By blocking PAF from binding to its receptor sites in the body, the ginkgolide B in ginkgo inhibits PAF-induced bronchoconstriction and airway hyperactivity. Ginkgo also contains antioxidant flavonoid compounds that may contribute to the herb's anti-inflammatory properties. As an antioxidant, ginkgo acts as a free radical scavenger and also inhibits oxidation of blood fats.

**Safety information:** *Ginkgo biloba* standardized extract is generally considered safe when used as directed. People using blood-thinning drugs (anticoagulants or antithrombotic agents) or supplements with blood-thinning effects should be cautious with ginkgo, as it may enhance the activity of these substances.

**Dosage advice:** Take 120–240 mg/day (capsules or liquid) in divided doses of standardized extract (50:1 concentrated extract standardized to 24 percent ginkgo flavone glycosides and 6 percent terpene lactones), or follow manufacturer's instructions. If using tincture, take 1–2 ml tincture mixed with 4 ounces of water three or four times daily.

## Glutathione

**Main action:** Antioxidant

Glutathione is a powerful antioxidant that is naturally produced by the liver. It functions as an electron donor and as such not only is it able to stabilize free radicals, but it also functions to keep vitamin C and other important antioxidant molecules working effectively as antioxidants. Considering the significant amount of oxidative damage that exists within the respiratory tissue of smokers and COPD patients, glutathione is an important supplement whose therapeutic value cannot be emphasized enough. Research substantiates the ability of glutathione to be beneficial in reversing the oxidant–antioxidant imbalances that occur in lung tissue as a result of the oxidative stress and inflammation associated with COPD.

Glutathione is produced mainly in the liver, utilizing three amino acids as building blocks: L-cysteine, glycine, and L-glutamate. Because it is a powerful antioxidant, glutathione is able to scavenge free radicals and support the antioxidant effects of other molecules, such as vitamin C.

For people with COPD, the preferred method for taking glutathione is by inhaling it through a nebulizer. Using this technique helps arrest the damage that is caused by free radicals. It stabilizes the lung tissue, halts oxidative stress, and facilitates the process of healing lung tissue. In order to take glutathione via your nebulizer, you will need a prescription for IV-grade reduced liquid glutathione. Liquid glutathione is not available at all pharmacies; it must usually be ordered from a compounding pharmacy.

If you are unable to obtain IV-grade reduced liquid glutathione for

---

### COPD Nebulizer Formula

This comprehensive nebulizer formula based on liquid glutathione helps ease COPD symptoms and heal damaged lung tissue. The combination of ingredients provides antioxidant, anti-inflammatory, antimicrobial, and expectorant actions. Because you must have a prescription for the first three ingredients, you will need to ask your doctor to order the formula for you from a compounding pharmacy. Compounding pharmacies specialize in custom-formulating medications for specific patient needs. Many compounding pharmacies offer mail-order services if you don't have a reliable compounding pharmacy in your area. (See appendix 1 for more information on working with compounding pharmacies.)

#### COPD Nebulizer Formula

| | |
|---|---|
| IV-grade reduced glutathione | 20 ml |
| IV-grade vitamin C | 8 ml |
| IV-grade 0.9% normal saline | 44 ml |
| Glycyrrhizic acid (liquid extract) | 20 ml |
| Children's Glycerite* (liquid extract) | 28 ml |

Dosage: 1–2 ml inhaled via nebulizer every three to four hours. Follow your doctor's instructions.

---

*Children's Glycerite is the trade name for a formula from Wise Woman Herbals in Oregon (see appendix 1 for contact information). Children's Glycerite is discussed in more detail on page 127 in chapter 7.

use in your nebulizer, oral glutathione can be taken either as straight glutathione or as a combination of the three amino acids the body needs to produce glutathione on its own. Research findings are somewhat divided as to which method of taking oral glutathione is best. Some evidence suggests that oral glutathione alone is poorly absorbed by the body; intake of the individual amino acids (L-cysteine, L-glutamate, and glycine) might be a more effective way to obtain adequate amounts of glutathione. As long as your liver is functioning properly, your body will make glutathione for you from these building blocks. (*Note:* If you are already taking oral N-acetylcysteine, you need not take any additional L-cysteine.)

**Dosage advice:** If using glutathione alone, take 600 mg daily. If using amino acid capsules or tablets, take 500–1,500 mg/day L-cysteine (only if not also taking NAC), 100–500 mg/day L-glutamate, and 500–1,000 mg/day glycine in divided doses.

**Safety information:** No adverse effects have been reported. Be sure to drink plenty of water when taking glutathione or its precursor amino acids to enhance absorption and uptake.

### Grape Seed Extract and Pycnogenol

**Main actions:** Antioxidant, anti-inflammatory

Both grape seed extract and Pycnogenol are rich in antioxidant compounds called oligomeric proanthocyanidins (OPCs), a type of flavonoid. Research suggests that OPCs may have significantly higher antioxidant activity than vitamin E and vitamin C. OPCs help protect against free radical damage throughout the body; they are able to support the immune system and moderate inflammatory responses. OPCs also work with glutathione in order to keep vitamin C functioning as an antioxidant. Additionally, according to laboratory studies, grape seed extract may have cancer-protective effects.

Pycnogenol is a trade name for an extract derived from the bark of the French maritime pine *(Pinus maritima)*. Research suggests that Pycnogenol can act as an anti-inflammatory agent, possibly due to its antioxidant capacity. Pycnogenol scavenges reactive oxygen and nitrogen species, as well as superoxide radicals, hydroxyl radicals, lipid peroxyl radicals, and peroxynitrite radicals. Pycnogenol may also inhibit the activation of several inflammatory mechanisms in the body. This may help reduce the inflammation experienced in COPD. In other laboratory studies, Pycnogenol has been shown to specifically inhibit smoking-induced platelet aggregation as well as protect against a tobacco-specific carcinogen known as NKK.

**Safety information:** No adverse effects have been reported.

**Dosage advice:** Take 50–200 mg daily (capsules or tablets).

## Hempseed Oil

**Main action:** Anti-inflammatory

Hempseed oil is an excellent source of essential fatty acids. Like flaxseed oil, it is one of the few plants that contain both omega-3 and omega-6 fatty acids. This essential fatty acid content suggests that it may be useful as an anti-inflammatory agent. Hempseed oil is obtained from the seeds of the cannabis plant *(Cannabis sativa),* but contains none of the psychoactive components of marijuana. Hempseed oil is sold as a nutritional supplement by several companies and is legal in all states. It has a natural nutty flavor that makes it very palatable. Try adding 1 to 2 tablespoons of hempseed oil per day to salads, cooked or raw vegetables, potatoes, pasta, or rice, or mix it with crushed garlic to make a dip for breads. Use it in marinades, salad dressings, cold or warm sauces, pâtés, and soups. You can also blend hempseed oil with fruit juices or smoothies.

Hempseed oil is a moderate source of omega-3 alpha-linolenic acid (ALA), a rich source of omega-6 linoleic acid (LA), and a moderate source of omega-6 gamma-linolenic acid (GLA).

**Safety information:** There have been occasional reports of nausea and diarrhea in people using hempseed oil. People with hemophilia and those using blood-thinning drugs (anticoagulants or antithrombotic agents) or supplements with blood-thinning effects should be cautious with hempseed oil, as it may enhance the activity of these substances. Hempseed oil should also be used cautiously in people diagnosed with breast or prostate cancer.

## Inosine

**Main actions:** Anti-inflammatory, immunomodulator

Inosine is popularly used as an endurance enhancer for athletes. There is no research evidence to support the use of inosine as an endurance enhancer; however, laboratory research suggests that inosine may act as an anti-inflammatory and an immunomodulator.

Inosine is found in a variety of plant and animal sources. It has been shown to inhibit pro-inflammatory cytokines.

**Dosage advice:** Take 1,000–5,000 mg daily in tablet or capsule form. Do not exceed 5,000 mg/day unless directed to do so by your physician.

## Lactoferrin

**Main action:** Antimicrobial

Lactoferrin is an amino acid that transports iron throughout the body. Because lactoferrin has a high affinity for iron, it readily attaches itself to iron molecules, effectively denying harmful bacteria the iron they need to grow and sustain themselves. This is what gives lactoferrin its natural antibiotic properties, making it useful during an acute respiratory tract infection.

Lactoferricin, a compound formed when the body breaks down lactoferrin, also has the ability to inhibit the activity of viruses and may help prevent the entry of viruses into normal cells.

**Dosage advice:** Take 250 mg daily (capsules).

**Safety information:** No adverse effects have been reported.

## Lipotropic Factors

**Main actions:** Liver support

Lipotropic factors promote improved liver function and fat metabolism by enhancing the flow of bile and fat to and from the liver. Most major manufacturers of dietary supplements offer lipotropic factor formulas. Good formulas contain choline, methionine, betaine, folic acid, and vitamins $B_6$ and $B_{12}$.

**Dosage advice:** Follow manufacturer's instructions.

**Safety information:** Lipotropic factors are generally considered safe. Refer to the label for any special precautions.

## Magnesium

**Main action:** Bronchodilator

How magnesium acts as a bronchodilator is not fully understood, but there is research and epidemiological data to support the use of magnesium in COPD. Magnesium has been demonstrated to relax smooth muscle, a finding that clearly indicates its potential usefulness as a bronchodilator. (Magnesium in intravenous form is used in some hospitals as a bronchodilator.) The relaxation of the smooth muscle surrounding the bronchi and bronchioles enables these airways to expand, which allows for greater airflow and ease in breathing.

**Dosage advice:** Take 350–500 mg daily (tablets or capsules). Do not exceed 500 mg/day without consulting your physician. Use a chelated magnesium formulation.

**Safety information:** Nausea and diarrhea are possible adverse reactions; these can be avoided by taking magnesium with food. Pregnant women and nursing mothers should not exceed 350 mg of supplemental magnesium daily unless directed by a physician. People with kidney failure or atrioventricular block (a serious heart problem) should avoid magnesium. People diagnosed with myasthenia gravis should also avoid supplemental magnesium.

## Manganese

**Main action:** Anti-inflammatory

Manganese is an essential trace mineral required for many of the body's functions. In particular, it serves as a cofactor for many classes of enzymes—those enzymes that can act only if they are bound to manganese. A limited amount of research suggests that manganese may have anti-inflammatory effects because of an ability to inhibit the activity of phospholipase $A_2$. Zinc is believed to work in a similar way (see page 123). Manganese is also required for the body to synthesize superoxide dimutase, a powerful antioxidant. Based on this research evidence, and the fact that zinc and manganese are not harmful supplements under normal conditions, it is reasonable to see if they will help in your particular case.

**Safety information:** No adverse effects have been reported at recommended dosages. People with liver problems, particularly liver failure, should not use manganese. Pregnant women and nursing mothers should not exceed 5 mg daily. The absorption of manganese may be decreased if it is taken at the same time as antacids, laxatives, tetracycline, calcium, iron, or magnesium.

**Dosage advice:** Take 2–10 mg daily (tablets or capsules).

## Milk Thistle Seed Extract

**Main actions:** Antioxidant, liver protective

Milk thistle seed *(Silybum marianum)* is one of the most important dietary supplements for liver support and protection. Considering the central role the liver plays as the body's major detoxifying organ, milk thistle is an important herb for COPD. People with COPD should take extra care to protect the liver because of all the extra stress caused by the toxins in cigarette smoke and medications, not to mention the effects of poor diet on liver health.

The efficacy of milk thistle seed extract is well established in the scientific research literature. Results of this research demonstrate that a standardized extract made from the seeds of the milk thistle plant has antioxidant and liver-protective effects. Standardized milk thistle extract contains a group of flavonoid compounds collectively known as silymarin. By acting as an antioxidant, silymarin protects the liver and enhances the liver's ability to process drugs, chemical pollutants, and other toxins.

Silymarin protects liver cells from toxins by increasing the liver's production of the all-important antioxidant glutathione. It also enhances the liver's ability to regenerate healthy cells. Silymarin exerts a wide variety of other liver-protective properties through its actions upon both liver cells and Kupffer cells, which are specialized macrophages (immune cells) within the liver. Silymarin inhibits the formation of leukotrienes by Kupffer cells, which helps to reduce inflammation in the liver. In addition, silymarin decreases the production of nitric oxide and superoxide anion radicals by Kupffer cells. Nitric oxide and superoxide anion radicals serve a limited purpose as part of the macrophage's process of killing pathogens, and are otherwise relatively harmless. However, these free radicals can lead to oxidative damage because they can readily react to form other free radicals, such as hydroxyl radicals, which are very dangerous to cells.

**Safety information:** Milk thistle is generally considered safe when used as directed. Except for occasional loose stools, no adverse effects have been reported.

**Dosage advice:** Take 140–420 mg daily (divided into two or three doses) of milk thistle extract standardized to 80 percent silymarin (capsules or tablets). If using tincture, take 1–2 ml mixed with 4 ounces of water or juice, two or three times daily.

## N-Acetylcysteine (NAC)

**Main actions:** Antioxidant, mucolytic

N-acetylcysteine (NAC) is the dietary supplement form of acetylcysteine, which is available only with a prescription. NAC capsule or tablet supplements are taken orally, while prescription acetylcysteine is a liquid that is used in the nebulizer.

The use of acetylcysteine in COPD is very well established in the scientific literature. It helps break up mucus and enables easier expectoration. Acetylcysteine acts as both an antioxidant and a mucolytic (a substance that breaks up mucus). As a mucolytic, acetylcysteine has direct effects on breaking the bonds between portions of the molecules that hold mucus together and thereby effectively reduces the viscosity (thickness) of mucus secretions. L-cysteine, an amino acid that is a major component of acetylcysteine, is one of the precursors of glutathione, a powerful antioxidant produced by the liver.

There is disagreement among experts as to which form of acetylcysteine—prescription or dietary supplement—better confers the mucolytic benefit. The fact is both routes of administration may be used simultaneously, but with care and the guidance of a physician. It is important to drink plenty of water and remain well hydrated when using acetylcysteine in any form. Follow the guidelines given at the end of chapter 4 to determine how much water you should be drinking every day.

**Safety information:** Nausea, vomiting, diarrhea, headache, and rashes are possible side effects. People with a history of peptic ulcer disease should use NAC cautiously. Individuals using nitrates may experience headaches if using NAC at the same time. NAC may reduce serum levels of carbamazepine (an epilepsy drug) in patients taking this drug.

**Dosage advice:** Take 600–1,200 mg one to three times daily (capsules or tablets) on an empty stomach. For better absorption, take with 50 mg vitamin $B_6$ and 100 mg vitamin C. (If using liquid acetylcysteine, follow your doctor's orders.)

## Oregano Essential Oil

**Main actions:** Anti-inflammatory, antimicrobial, expectorant

The essential oil of oregano contains the compound carvacrol, which is known to have antimicrobial properties. This makes oregano essential oil useful in treating some of the respiratory infections that are often troublesome for people with COPD. Oregano helps reduce inflammation in the mucous membranes of the bronchial passages, and, as an expectorant, also helps clear the bronchial passages of mucus.

It is very important to check the label of the product you purchase to be sure its main ingredient is carvacrol, not thymol.

**Safety information:** Essential oils are much more concentrated and thus more potentially dangerous than herbs and herb extracts. They should be used in dilution and not taken internally unless one is very sure about product quality. As noted above, it is essential that carvacrol (not thymol) is the main ingredient in the oregano essential oil product you use. Oregano essential oil high in thymol is not considered safe for therapeutic use.

Do not exceed a total daily dosage (taken orally or inhaled) of $2^1/_2$ ml (about 70 drops) oregano essential oil without consulting your health care professional. Pregnant women should not use oregano essential oil.

**Dosage advice:** Oregano essential oil can be taken orally or inhaled using a steam inhalation device or nebulizer. The Vicks Vaposteam Inhaler is a good choice for a compact yet effective and inexpensive steam inhalation device.

To take orally, mix $^1/_2$ ml (14 drops) with 2 ounces of water and drink one or two times daily.

To make a steam inhalation, mix 1 ml (about 28 drops) with 2 to 3 ounces of very hot (but not boiling) water in a steam inhaler one or two times daily.

To take via a nebulizer, mix $^3/_4$ ml (21 drops) mixed with 2 ml of warm distilled water and inhale one or two times daily.

## Quercetin

**Main actions:** Antioxidant, anti-inflammatory, immunomodulator

Quercetin is a type of natural antioxidant that belongs to a large class of chemical compounds called flavonoids. Good food sources of quercetin are apples, onions, black and green tea, and grapefruit, but it is difficult to get therapeutic amounts of quercetin from the diet. This means that in order to get a therapeutic effect from quercetin, it may be best to take a supplement.

Research indicates that quercetin has anti-inflammatory and anti-oxidant effects and acts as an immunomodulator (a substance that has effects on the immune system). Quercetin's anti-inflammatory properties are related at least in part to its ability to inhibit lipoxygenase, the enzyme necessary for the formation of pro-inflammatory leukotriene $B_4$ ($LTB_4$). Research also indicates that quercetin can inhibit the formation of pro-inflammatory series-2 prostaglandins. Other studies have shown that quercetin inhibits the activity of cells (mast cells, basophils, and neutrophils) that promote inflammation, lending further scientific support for quercetin's anti-inflammatory and immunomodulating activities. As quercetin's inhibition of lipoxygenase limits the formation of all series-4 leukotrienes, quercetin can also aid in lessening bronchoconstriction.

**Dosage advice:** Take 500 mg (capsules or tablets) three times daily. Absorption of quercetin is believed to be enhanced by bromelain and papain (digestive enzymes derived from papaya).

**Safety information:** There have been rare reports of nausea, headache, and mild tingling in the extremities in people taking quercetin supplements. People taking quinolone antibiotics or cisplatin (a cancer chemotherapy drug) should not take quercetin supplements.

## Selenium

**Main action:** Antioxidant

Selenium is a trace mineral used by the body to produce glutathione peroxidase, which functions as a natural antioxidant. The selenium-dependent glutathione peroxidases help prevent oxidative damage to cell membranes and DNA. Because people with COPD tend to have oxidative damage to their lungs and may be at higher risk for lung cancer, by reducing the concentrations of reactive oxygen in cells, particularly those of the respiratory epithelium, glutathione peroxidases play a key role in helping to protect the respiratory epithelium (lung cells) and DNA from oxidative damage.

**Safety information:** No adverse events have been reported at the recommended dosages. Pregnant women and nursing mothers should not exceed 400 mcg daily.

**Dosage advice:** Take 50–400 mcg daily. Do not exceed 400 mcg daily without the guidance of a physician.

## Serrapeptase

**Main actions:** Anti-inflammatory, mucolytic

Serrapeptase, also known as serratiopeptidase, is a well-researched enzyme that has been shown to have anti-inflammatory and mucolytic effects, suggesting that it might be helpful in emphysema, chronic bronchitis, and bronchiectasis. By digesting (dissolving) nonliving tissue such as blood clots and arterial plaques, as well as reducing neutrophils, serrapeptase reduces the inflammation that is associated with COPD and helps with cardiovascular disease. Serrapeptase also enhances mucus clearance by thinning sputum.

Serrapeptase has been researched and used clinically (mostly in Europe and Japan) for more than twenty-five years. Serrapeptase was first isolated from a naturally occurring bacterium found in the intestine of the silkworm. Today the enzyme is produced commercially through a special fermentation process.

**Safety information:** Serrapeptase is generally considered quite safe. There have been a few reports in which the use of serrapeptase was suspected of causing either pneumonitis (inflammation of lung tissue) or dermatitis. Discuss the use of this supplement with your physician.

**Dosage advice:** Take 20,000–60,000 IU (international units) one to three times a day, or follow your physician's instructions. Do not exceed 180,000 IU a day without consulting your physician. Take on an empty stomach.

## Superoxide Dismutase

**Main action:** Antioxidant

Superoxide dimutase (SOD) is the name given to a class of enzymes that are produced by the body in order to protect cells from oxidative damage. SOD neutralizes free radicals, particularly the superoxide radicals, by converting them into hydrogen peroxide and molecular oxygen. The ability of SOD to neutralize superoxide radicals, which are the most common free radicals in the body, is beneficial in addressing the oxidative damage in lung tissue.

**Safety information:** SOD is generally considered safe. Refer to the label for any special precautions.

**Dosage advice:** Take 2,000 MF units (McCord-Fridovich units) in tablet form one to three times daily between meals.

## Vitamin A

**Main action:** Immunomodulator, promotes healthy mucous membranes in the respiratory tract, general health benefits

Vitamin A is an essential vitamin that the body needs for proper function. Adequate amounts of vitamin A are needed for proper immune function, to help prevent infection, and to support pulmonary function. The body makes vitamin A out of beta-carotene consumed in the diet. Sometimes, however, the amount of vitamin A formed from dietary beta-carotene is not enough for therapeutic benefits and supplemental vitamin A is necessary.

**Safety information:** Do not exceed 25,000 IU a day without consulting your physician. Vitamin A is a fat-soluble vitamin that is not as readily metabolized as are water-soluble vitamins.

**Dosage advice:** Take 25,000 IU daily.

## B-complex Vitamins

**Main actions:** Enhance tissue repair and healing, general health benefits

The B vitamins serve as constituent components for more than one hundred enzymes. In order for these enzymes to properly perform their functions, many of which involve healing and tissue repair, an adequate amount of B vitamins is necessary.

**Safety information:** B vitamins are generally considered safe. Refer to the label for any special precautions.

**Dosage advice:** Follow instructions on the product label.

## Vitamin C

**Main actions:** Antioxidant, immunomodulator, enhances tissue repair and healing, general health benefits

Vitamin C is one of the most important antioxidants in existence. It is capable of reducing reactive oxygen species (oxygen free radicals) as well as reactive nitrogen compounds. Vitamin C also helps to maintain cellular concentrations of reduced glutathione, another extremely important antioxidant.

As an antioxidant, vitamin C protects the bronchial airways from oxidative stress that can lead to bronchoconstriction. It is also helpful in counteracting the oxidative damage brought about through smoking. Vitamin C also enhances immune function, acts as an anti-inflammatory by reducing histamine levels, and aids in the healing of inflamed tissue. Because vitamin C is involved in the biosynthesis of elastin, the principal protein molecule that comprises the elastic fibers within the interalveolar septum (alveolar wall), it helps to repair damaged lung tissue.

I recommend vitamin C formulations that contain bioflavonoids, including rutin. Bioflavonoids greatly improve the body's ability to absorb and utilize vitamin C.

**Safety information:** High doses of vitamin C can cause nausea, diarrhea, and flatulence. If any of these side effects occur, simply cut back the amount of vitamin C you are taking. These are the side effects of reaching what is called bowel tolerance—the maximum amount of vitamin C you can take without experiencing stomach upset. People taking cancer chemotherapy drugs should consult their doctors before taking supplemental vitamin C.

**Dosage advice:** Take 1,000 mg every two to three hours to bowel tolerance (see safety information) up to a total of 6,000–10,000 mg/day. For better absorption, use a buffered form of vitamin C that also contains calcium and magnesium.

## Vitamin E

**Main actions:** Antioxidant, general health benefits

Vitamin E (also known by its chemical name, d-alpha-tocopherol) is a powerful antioxidant, which makes it quite useful in counteracting the oxidative damage that exists in the lungs. Vitamin E also has other clearly established health benefits that make it an appropriate supplement for general health maintenance. Like selenium, the body uses vitamin E in the formation of glutathione peroxidases.

In terms of reducing inflammation related to COPD, scientific research indicates that vitamin E and vitamin E analogs (slightly modified forms of vitamin E) are inhibitors of phospholipase $A_2$. By inhibiting the release of arachidonic acid, vitamin E inhibits the formation of pro-inflammatory series-4 leukotrienes and series-2 prostaglandins. This implies that vitamin E may help reduce the inflammation and broncho-constriction associated with COPD.

**Safety information:** Do not exceed 1,600 IU/day of vitamin E unless under the advice of a physician. People with a history of bleeding disorders, hemorrhagic stroke, hemophilia, or vitamin K deficiency should use vitamin E with extreme caution. In addition, those using blood-thinning drugs (anticoagulants or antithrombotic agents) or supplements with blood-thinning effects should be cautious with vitamin E, as it may enhance the activity of these substances.

**Dosage advice:** Take 400 IU three or four times daily (tablets or capsules). Take with 50 to 100 mg vitamin C in order to enhance absorption. Higher doses of vitamin E may be needed for therapeutic benefit; however, do not exceed 1,600 IU daily without your physician's recommendation and supervision.

## Zinc

**Main actions:** Immunomodulator, anti-inflammatory, general health benefits

Zinc is an essential mineral that is involved in myriad biochemical reactions in the body. As it pertains to COPD, though, there is research to suggest that zinc can inhibit phospholipase $A_2$. By inhibiting phospholipase $A_2$, zinc may contribute to lessening the release of arachidonic acid, which decreases the formation of pro-inflammatory series-4 leukotrienes and series-2 prostaglandins. Although more research is needed, it is reasonable to think that this effect could contribute to reducing inflammation and bronchoconstriction.

Zinc also enhances the function of the immune system.

**Safety information:** Nausea, vomiting, metallic taste, headache, or drowsiness may occur at doses higher than 30 mg/day. Do not take zinc at the same time as quinolone antibiotics or tetracycline, as this may decrease the absorption of both the antibiotics and the zinc. Pregnant or nursing women should not exceed 15 mg/day of zinc.

**Dosage advice:** Take 50 mg two or three times daily (in tablets or capsules).

# Herbal Medicine

Herbs have been an integral part of the healing arts since the dawn of civilization. For thousands of years, essentially every known culture that has ever inhabited planet Earth has used herbs medicinally. The medicinal use of many herbs today is still based upon their historically demonstrated effects, but ongoing scientific analysis and research on the medicinal effects of herbs is confirming the observations of traditional herbalists throughout history. Researchers are also discovering new applications and shedding light on the many roles herbs play in human health. Perhaps the most significant benefit of this research is that it has begun to provide scientific explanations for the actions of many herbs.

Current scientific research methods are absolutely necessary in order to advance our understanding of science and medicine, and double-blind clinical studies certainly yield much-needed data concerning a substance's effectiveness and safety. However, we would be remiss to disregard the wisdom and knowledge of medicinal herbs collected by various cultures throughout history, if only because many valuable herbs have not yet been subjected to current research methods or double-blind clinical studies.

Learn as much as you can about herbs. They will be an important factor in your healing process. When we think of herbs, we often forget they are plant foods that also provide a whole spectrum of nutrients that complement and support the healing process. Working with a skilled practitioner who not only knows the nuances of your condition but is also well versed in the use of herbs will in all likelihood enable you to efficiently determine which herbs will benefit your condition.

I believe that if an herb has been consistently and reliably used over the centuries based on well-recognized medicinal properties, this constitutes historical proof of an herb's effectiveness. I would further submit that using the historical record of an herb to substantiate its medicinal value is every bit as legitimate as using a modern double-blind clinical study. Passing the test of traditional use over time, rather than clinical trials, provides the most useful information about how to use any particular herb safely, effectively, and appropriately.

Herbs, in general, are quite safe when used properly. This does not mean that they never cause side effects, but when properly administered, side effects are rare and significantly less serious than the common side effects of most pharmaceutical medications. Do not exceed recommended dosages. If you are pregnant, nursing, or taking pharmaceutical medications, consult your doctor before using an herb.

## THE USE OF HERBS IN COPD

The value of herbs as part of a complete holistic approach to address the issues of COPD is incalculable. Within the context of an approach that is always grounded in the dietary and nutritional approaches that were covered in chapter 5, not only can herbs be used to address the main symptomatic issues of COPD, but they also work synergistically to help bring about overall healing and restoration of health to the extent that is possible.

The herbs that I have chosen to include in this chapter all have a well-established traditional basis for use in COPD. Although most herbs usually have multiple actions that work together, I focus on the actions that are immediately relevant to COPD. All of the herbs described here, with the exception of olive leaf, are indicated to be used orally as either a liquid extract (tincture) or an infusion ("herbal tea"). Olive leaf should be taken by capsule because this is the most readily available form of olive leaf. In general, however, liquid extracts are easier for the body to assimilate than are capsules.

You may have to try several herbs or herbal tea combinations before finding those that work most effectively for you. This is one of the reasons I list forty-five herbs overall and provide ten herbal tea combinations in this chapter. As you learn more about herbs, you will be better able to fine-tune your choices to select herbs that will provide you with the most benefit for your particular case.

A liquid herbal formula that I have found to be particularly helpful for easing respiratory symptoms is Children's Glycerite, from Wise Woman Herbals, in Oregon (see appendix 1 for contact information). Children's Glycerite is part of the COPD nebulizer formula that was discussed in the last chapter, but it is presented again here as it is also quite useful as a tincture taken orally. Children's Glycerite liquid extract is formulated according to traditional herbal principles to help with respiratory symptoms and, despite its name, is appropriate for use by adults. The formula contains echinacea, wild cherry bark, yerba santa, elecampane, goldenseal, osha, mullein, ginger, and bitter orange essential oil in a base of vegetable glycerine. Mix 20 to 60 drops (1–2 ml) in a glass of water and take one to four times a day.

Contact information for other reputable suppliers of herbal extracts and bulk herbs can be found in appendix 1.

## WORKING WITH HERBS

Working with herbs may take some getting used to in the beginning, but it can become an enjoyable process, especially when it comes to using bulk herbs to prepare formulas for herbal tea combinations. You may want to consult a book on herbal medicine–making to learn more about this ancient craft. See appendix 2 for suggestions.

### Herbal Terminology

To help you get started with herbs, there are a few terms you should understand. A *tincture* is a kind of liquid herb extract usually prepared with alcohol and water. Liquid extracts that do not contain alcohol are also available. These nonalcoholic extracts are usually prepared with vegetable glycerin and are suitable for individuals who cannot tolerate alcohol.

A *standardized extract* is a highly processed herb extract that is guaranteed to contain a certain amount of specific chemical compounds believed to contribute to the herb's activities. (Because such extracts are highly processed and more like drugs than traditional herbal formulas, I discussed the use of standardized milk thistle and *Ginkgo biloba* extracts in chapter 6, with other dietary supplements.)

An *infusion* is a water-based herbal extract of leaves and flowers, commonly known as an "herbal tea." An infusion is prepared by steeping the leaves or flowers in boiling water. Pour 1 pint of boiling water over $1/2$ to 1 ounce of the dried herb in a pot made of enamel, porcelain, or glass. The dried herb may be in a tea bag, a tea ball, or loose. Allow the mixture to steep for about 10 minutes. Strain and drink lukewarm. A little bit of honey may be added if necessary to improve the taste.

Another kind of herbal tea, made by simmering roots, bark, or other tough material, is called a *decoction*. To prepare a decoction, boil about $1/2$ ounce of herb (roots, bark, or seeds) per cup of water in a glass pot for about 10 minutes and then allow to steep, covered, for an additional 3 to 5 minutes. Strain and drink lukewarm. As with infusions, a little bit of honey may be added if necessary to improve the taste.

According to classical medicine-making techniques, most roots, barks, and seeds should be prepared as decoctions (by simmering) as opposed to infusion (by steeping). The exceptions are volatile oil–rich roots like valerian. Volatile oil–rich infusions (containing herbs like thyme and many other plants in the mint family) should be covered while steeping to prevent loss of the volatile oils.

Recipes for herbal formulas are often given in terms of a measurement called a *part*. A part can be any amount you choose, depending on the size of the batch you are making. Parts simply represent a ratio. Here's an example. If you decide 1 part is 1 cup, then a recipe that calls for 1 part peppermint, 2 parts chamomile, and 1 part nettle leaf will contain 1 cup peppermint, 2 cups chamomile, and 1 cup nettle leaf—a total of 4 cups of formula.

When determining dosages of tinctures and liquid extracts, note that 1 milliliter (ml) is approximately 28 drops. One ounce is approximately equivalent to 30 ml.

## TABLE 8. HERBAL ACTIONS RELEVANT TO COPD

| Action | Effect |
| --- | --- |
| Anti-inflammatory | Decreases underlying inflammation |
| Antimicrobial (including antibacterial, antifungal, and antiviral) | Kills organisms that can cause infections |
| Antioxidant | Helps heal and protect against oxidative damage (see chapter 6 for more details) |
| Antispasmodic | Relieves muscular spasms |
| Antitussive | Relieves coughing |
| Astringent | Tones and tightens tissues; dries excess secretions |
| Bronchodilator | Helps relax bronchial smooth muscle so the bronchi and bronchioles can expand |
| Demulcent | Provides a soothing coating for irritated tissue |
| Diaphoretic | Promotes perspiration |
| Expectorant | Makes it easier to expel mucus from the respiratory passages |
| Immunomodulator | Affects the function of the immune system |
| Sedative | Calming to the nervous system (may also be called a nervine) |
| Tonic | Helps heal and support the function and structure of tissues or organs |

## THE HERBS

The descriptions that follow explain traditional herb uses most relevant to COPD. When possible, I have also presented current scientific research findings to further substantiate the actions and use of the herbs.

This is just a brief introduction to some of the many actions of these herbs. Many wonderful books devoted to herbal medicine explain these and other herb effects in greater detail. I've included some suggestions for additional reading in appendix 2.

### Astragalus *(Astragalus membranaceous)*

**Main actions:** Antiviral, antioxidant, immunomodulator, tonic
**Part used:** Dried root

Astragalus is an important herb in traditional Chinese medicine (TCM). It is helpful in fighting infections of the mucous membranes, especially the mucous membranes of the respiratory tract. Astragalus is also an excellent tonic for strengthening the lungs and for combating the debility and wasting that often accompany COPD. Astragalus has also been shown to inhibit lipid peroxidation, making it useful as an antioxidant.

**Safety information:** No adverse effects have been reported. Do not use astragalus if you have a fever.

**Dosage advice:** Take 1–2 ml tincture mixed with 4 ounces of water three or four times daily.

### Cayenne *(Capsicum annuum)*

**Main actions:** Antimicrobial, circulatory stimulant, expectorant
**Part used:** Ripe fruit

Cayenne pepper, made from ripe chili peppers, is useful as an expectorant to help expel the thick mucus secretions that are characteristic of COPD.

Cayenne also acts as a stimulant to enhance blood circulation. Because of this ability to enhance circulation, cayenne is often added to formulas with other herbs to enhance their absorption and effectiveness. Cayenne also contains compounds, called capsaicinoids, that have been shown in laboratory research to have antimicrobial effects against *Streptococcus pyogenes* bacteria.

**Safety information:** Cayenne is generally considered safe when used as recommended.

**Dosage advice:** Take 1 ml tincture mixed with 4 ounces of water or juice three to five times daily.

## Echinacea *(Echinacea purpurea, E. angustifolia, E. pallida)*

**Main actions:** Anti-inflammatory, immunomodulator, protects collagen
**Parts used:** Fresh root, leaves, and flowers

Echinacea has a number of actions that make it appropriate for people with COPD. Echinacea is perhaps best known as an immunomodulator, a substance that enhances the ability of the immune system to fight off infection. Studies show that echinacea stimulates the activity of macrophages, granulocytes, and leukocytes, immune cells that attack and destroy disease-causing microbes. The herb seems especially helpful for infections of the respiratory tract. In clinical research, echinacea reduced the severity of respiratory tract infections and shortened the duration of symptoms.

Laboratory research has shown that echinacea enhances the ability of leukocytes to kill *Staphylococcus* bacteria (commonly called staph). This is an important capability, insofar as many COPD patients have tested positive for MRSA (methicillin-resistant *Staphylococcus aureus*), an antibiotic-resistant strain of staphylococcus. *S. aureus* is often the pathogenic culprit involved in the recurrent episodes of pneumonia that are experienced by individuals with COPD. Because of *Staphylococcus aureus'* resistance to antibiotics, an episode of pneumonia due to *S. aureus* can be particularly serious for a COPD patient. Echinacea should therefore always be considered in the treatment strategy for an *S. aureus*–related infection for its ability to boosting the infection-fighting capacity of the immune system.

Laboratory research has also shown that echinacea can help protect the integrity of collagen (an important component of the connective tissue that makes up many body structures). This action may be due to echinacea's content of caffeic acid derivatives known as echinacosides. These compounds have been shown to protect type-III collagen from oxidative damage caused by free radicals. Because type-III collagen is one of the components of the interalveolar septum, echinacea may be able to help maintain the structural integrity of the acinus and promote the healing of damaged tissue.

Laboratory studies also suggest that echinacea acts as an anti-inflammatory through effects upon cyclooxygenase and 5-lipoxygenase. By inhibiting cyclooxygenase and 5-lipoxygenase, echinacea may reduce the formation of pro-inflammatory series-4 leukotrienes and series-2 prostaglandins. This may contribute to lessening inflammation in the bronchial walls, opening the airway, and reducing mucus production.

**Safety information:** Echinacea is generally considered safe when used as directed.

**Dosage advice:** Take 2 ml tincture mixed with 4 ounces of water three to six times daily. In cases of severe infection, take up to 4 ml every one to two hours until the infection abates.


## Elecampane *(Inula helenium)*

**Main actions:** Antimicrobial, expectorant, respiratory tonic
**Parts used:** Root (rhizome) and flower

Elecampane is useful for reducing the excessive mucus secretions and wet, productive coughs that are often characteristic of chronic bronchitis. Elecampane also soothes irritated mucous membranes in the respiratory tract. The herb contains compounds called sesquiterpene lactones that have demonstrated antimicrobial activity, including antibacterial and antifungal actions, in laboratory studies.

**Safety information:** Pregnant women should avoid elecampane.

**Dosage advice:** Take 1–2 ml tincture mixed with 4 ounces of water three to five times daily.

## Garlic *(Allium sativum)*

**Main actions:** Antimicrobial, antiviral, antioxidant, lipid-lowering
**Part used:** Fresh whole bulb

Among its many medicinal applications, garlic has been used historically to treat infections and inflammation and to clear mucus from the respiratory tract. Fresh raw garlic has a long history of traditional use as a treatment for respiratory tract infections, including those associated with bronchitis. In laboratory studies, garlic has demonstrated an ability to kill many microorganisms, including *Staphylococcus* and *Streptococcus* bacteria as well as several viruses.

Garlic also has antioxidant properties; research has shown that it increases intracellular levels of reduced glutathione, which prevents free radicals from indiscriminately stealing electrons from cell membranes or other molecules. Garlic's antioxidant capabilities are further enhanced, as it also contains the important antioxidant selenium. Although not directly related to COPD, garlic's well-established ability to lower total serum cholesterol as well as low-density lipoprotein cholesterol (LDL or "bad" cholesterol) is a positive health benefit not to be ignored.

**Safety information:** Garlic may cause stomach upset in sensitive individuals, including nursing babies. People using blood-thinning drugs (anticoagulants or antithrombotic agents) or supplements with blood-thinning effects should be cautious with garlic, as it may enhance the activity of these substances.

**Dosage advice:** Take 2 ml tincture mixed with 4 ounces of water or juice two or three times daily.

### Ginger *(Zingiber officinale)*

**Main actions:** Anti-inflammatory, diaphoretic, expectorant
**Part used:** Root

Ginger is perhaps best known for its ability to enhance digestion and to relieve nausea, vomiting, indigestion, and gas. Ginger is also a traditional remedy in formulas for coughs and colds in TCM and other traditional medicine systems. In addition, research has shown that ginger has anti-inflammatory properties. In laboratory studies, ginger inhibited 5-lipoxygenase and cyclooxygenase, an effect that reduces the formation of series-4 leukotrienes and pro-inflammatory series-2 prostaglandins. With a reduction in leukotrienes and pro-inflammatory prostaglandins, there will be a consequent reduction in inflammation and bronchoconstriction. Ginger has also been used as an expectorant and to relieve shortness of breath.

**Safety information:** Ginger is generally considered safe when used as recommended.

**Dosage advice:** Take 1–2 ml tincture mixed with 4 ounces of water or juice three or four times daily.

### Ginkgo *(Ginkgo biloba)*

**Main actions:** Anti-inflammatory, antioxidant, enhances microcirculation (circulation of blood in tiny capillaries)
**Part used:** Leaf

Ginkgo has anti-inflammatory and antioxidant actions that make it useful in COPD. *Ginkgo biloba* standardized extract has been extensively studied for its ability to enhance peripheral blood circulation (circulation in tiny blood vessels), including circulation to the brain. See chapter 6 for a detailed discussion of the benefits of this herb.

**Safety information:** People using blood-thinning drugs (anticoagulants or antithrombotic agents) or supplements with blood-thinning effects should be cautious with ginkgo, as it may enhance the activity of these substances.

**Dosage advice:** Take 1–2 ml tincture mixed with 4 ounces of water three or four times daily. If using a standardized extract, the dosage is 120–240 mg/day in divided doses, or follow manufacturer's instructions.

## Ginseng *(Panax ginseng)*

**Main actions:** Rejuvenating tonic, antioxidant
**Part used:** Root

In traditional Chinese medicine, ginseng is a valuable tonic useful for helping people recover from debilitating illness. It is considered most appropriate for older people and for use during convalescence. As COPD is most often an affliction of middle-aged to elderly people, ginseng is quite useful in addressing the debility that is associated with COPD and aging. Ginseng strengthens the lungs and enhances both physical energy and mental acuity. Ginseng also exerts antioxidant effects through its ability to increase the activity of glutathione peroxidase in the liver. There is also some research that suggests that ginseng can stimulate the immune system.

**Safety information:** According to TCM, do not use ginseng if you have a fever or an acute infection. If you have heart disease or diabetes, consult your doctor before taking ginseng.

**Dosage advice:** Take 1–2 ml tincture mixed with 4 ounces of water two or three times daily.

## Goldenseal *(Hydrastis canadensis)*

**Main actions:** Astringent, antibacterial, anti-inflammatory
**Part used:** Root (rhizome)

Goldenseal has a drying and cleansing effect on mucous membranes. This astringent action makes it useful in addressing the chronic inflammation and excess mucus secretions characteristic of COPD. The herb has a traditional reputation for effectiveness against respiratory tract infections.

In laboratory studies, goldenseal has shown antimicrobial actions against *Streptococcus pyogenes* and *Staphylococcus aureus* bacteria. A combination of echinacea and goldenseal extracts is a traditional remedy that may help protect against pathogens involved in the recurrent respiratory infections that are characteristic of COPD.

**Safety information:** Goldenseal should be avoided by individuals with glucose-6-phosphate dehydrogenase deficiency (an inherited condition common in African Americans that causes the premature destruction of red blood cells when an affected individual is exposed to certain medications or chemicals, such as goldenseal, that cause oxidative stress). Goldenseal should be used only for a week or two at a time, as it can kill beneficial bacteria in the intestines.

**Dosage advice:** Take 1–2 ml tincture mixed with 4 ounces of water three or four times daily.

### Gumweed *(Grindelia camporum)*

**Main actions:** Antimicrobial, anti-inflammatory, expectorant
**Parts used:** Dried leaves and flowers

Commonly known as asthma weed, *Grindelia* has a traditional reputation for helping to ease bronchial irritation and the unproductive coughs associated with constricted airways and wheezing. Gumweed is also useful for upper respiratory tract infections. In laboratory studies, it has demonstrated antimicrobial activity as well as anti-inflammatory actions.

**Safety information:** Gumweed is generally considered safe when used as recommended.

**Dosage advice:** Take 1–2 ml tincture mixed with 4 ounces of water two to four times daily.

## Hyssop *(Hyssopus officinalis)*

**Main actions:** Antimicrobial, expectorant, can inhibit spasms
**Parts used:** Leaf and flower

As a well-established expectorant, hyssop has been used historically to help relieve mucus congestion in the lungs. Hyssop also contains compounds that are antimicrobial and antiviral.

**Safety information:** Hyssop is generally considered safe when used as directed. Do not use hyssop during pregnancy.

**Dosage advice:** Take 1–2 ml tincture mixed with 4 ounces of water two or three times daily.

## Licorice *(Glycyrrhiza glabra)*

**Main actions:** Anti-inflammatory, antiviral, expectorant
**Part used:** Root

Licorice has well-established anti-inflammatory properties. It has also demonstrated antiviral effects in laboratory studies. As an antiviral, licorice is effective against influenza infection, a feature that is beneficial for COPD patients. Licorice is soothing to the mucous membranes of the respiratory tract and is useful in clearing the phlegm associated with chronic bronchitis.

In laboratory studies, licorice has inhibited cyclooxygenase and lipoxygenase. Inhibition of these enzymes reduces the formation of series-4 leukotrienes and series-2 prostaglandins, which will lead to a reduction of the inflammation and bronchoconstriction in the bronchial walls.

**Safety information:** People with high blood pressure, diabetes, kidney problems, cirrhosis of the liver, and other liver disease should avoid using whole licorice root or licorice extracts containing glycyrrhizin. Do not take glycyrrhizin or whole licorice root extracts in combination with high blood pressure medications or laxatives. Excessive, long-term use of whole licorice or licorice extracts containing glycyrrhizin can result in high blood pressure; however, any elevation in blood pressure due to the herb will return to normal when use of the herb is stopped. Do not use licorice during pregnancy.

**Dosage advice:** Take 1–2 ml tincture mixed with 4 ounces of water three or four times daily.

## Marshmallow *(Althaea officinalis)*

**Main actions:** Anti-inflammatory, antioxidant, demulcent, expectorant
**Parts used:** Root, leaf

Marshmallow has a demulcent action that is very soothing to the mucous membranes of the respiratory tract. It is particularly helpful when bronchial irritation and inflammation are associated with a dry, unproductive cough. In laboratory studies, marshmallow has also exhibited strong antioxidant activity.

**Safety information:** Marshmallow is generally considered safe when it is used as recommended.

**Dosage advice:** Take 2–3 ml tincture mixed with 4 ounces of water three or four times daily.

## Milk Thistle *(Silybum marianum)*

**Main actions:** Antioxidant, liver protective
**Part used:** Seed

Milk thistle seed is an important herb for people with COPD because it helps counteract the stress the condition puts on the liver. Because the best-studied milk thistle extract is a highly processed standardized extract, milk thistle is covered in detail in chapter 6 with other dietary supplements.

**Safety information:** Milk thistle seed is generally considered safe when used as directed.

Dosage advice: Take 1–2 ml of tincture mixed with 4 ounces of water or juice two or three times daily. If using standardized extract, the dosage is 140–420 mg daily (divided into two or three doses) of milk thistle extract standardized to 80 percent silymarin (capsules or tablets).

## Mullein *(Verbascum thapsus)*

Main actions: Anti-inflammatory, demulcent, expectorant, respiratory tonic
Parts used: Leaf and flower

Mullein leaf has a long history of traditional use as a respiratory tract tonic and for the treatment of respiratory tract infections. Mullein, like marshmallow root, is very soothing to the mucous membranes of the respiratory tract. Mullein eases inflammation and has an expectorant effect on the phlegm associated with chronic bronchitis.

Safety information: Mullein is generally considered safe when used as recommended.

Dosage advice: Take 2–3 ml tincture mixed with 4 ounces of water three or four times daily.

## Myrrh *(Commiphora molmol)*

Main actions: Anti-inflammatory, antimicrobial, expectorant
Part used: Resin

Although myrrh is best known as an ingredient for incense, its medicinal use for COPD is well substantiated. Myrrh is particularly useful in cases of chronic bronchitis where the mucous membranes have become sluggish and there is excessive and persistent mucus, and in cases of bronchiectasis, in which green sputum often indicates the presence of stagnant pus. Whether it is from chronic inflammation or infection, whenever there is excessive and tenacious mucus in the respiratory tract, myrrh should be considered as part of the therapeutic protocol.

**Safety information:** Myrrh is generally considered safe when used as directed. Pregnant women should avoid myrrh.

**Dosage advice:** Take 1–2 ml tincture mixed with 4 ounces of water two to four times daily.

## Osha *(Ligusticum porterii)*

**Main actions:** Anti-inflammatory, antimicrobial, expectorant
**Part used:** Root

Osha root is a traditional Native American remedy with a long history of use for treating respiratory conditions and inflammation. Osha root has expectorant, antimicrobial, and anti-inflammatory properties that make it particularly useful for COPD. It is well suited for most infections of the respiratory tract, especially those that are viral in origin. It is effective for bronchial inflammation and helps bring up respiratory mucus secretions. Because it also has the ability to relax bronchial smooth muscle, osha helps to ease breathing by lessening bronchoconstriction. Osha also induces sweating and helps eliminate toxins through the pores of the skin.

**Safety information:** Pregnant women should avoid osha.

**Dosage advice:** Take 1–2 ml tincture mixed with 4 ounces of water three or four times daily.

## Thyme *(Thymus officinalis)*

**Main actions:** Antimicrobial, expectorant, bronchial antispasmodic
**Parts used:** Leaf and flower

Thyme can help alleviate the bronchial spasms that so often accompany the coughing caused by COPD. Thyme is also quite useful for treating the inflammation and excess mucus secretions commonly associated with COPD. Thyme stimulates cilia so that they are better able to perform their function of sweeping away mucus secretions, and has strong antibacterial effects.

**Safety information:** Thyme is generally considered safe when it is used as recommended.

**Dosage advice:** Take 1–2 ml tincture mixed with 4 ounces of water three or four times daily.


## Valerian *(Valeriana officinalis)*

**Main actions:** Sedative, antispasmodic
**Part used:** Root

Valerian has a strong traditional reputation for effectiveness as an herbal sedative, useful for calming the nerves and relieving anxiety and insomnia. People with COPD can become anxious and excitable when experiencing shortness of breath (dyspnea). During an episode of acute dyspnea, valerian can help the sufferer relax and remain calm while efforts are taken to ease his or her breathing. Although exactly how valerian works remains an active area of study, some researchers believe valerian's sedative effects may be related to its content of valerenic acid, a chemical compound. Studies show that valerenic acid slows the breakdown of GABA, an important neurotransmitter (a chemical messenger in the brain). GABA acts to inhibit the flow of nerve trasmission from one nerve to the next, which has a relaxing effect on the body. It is believed that increasing the availability of GABA is what gives valerian its sedative properties.

**Safety information:** Valerian is generally considered safe when used as directed.

**Dosage advice:** Take 1–2 ml tincture mixed with 2 ounces of water as needed.


## White Horehound *(Marrubium vulgare)*

**Main actions:** Antimicrobial, antispasmodic, expectorant
**Parts used:** Leaf and flower

Horehound has a long history of use for respiratory tract infections, especially bronchitis. It has been traditionally used to treat inflammation of the mucous membranes in the respiratory tract accompanied by an increase in mucus flow. This herb is considered especially helpful for nonproductive coughs. In laboratory studies, white horehound has shown antimicrobial actions, including effects against both viruses and bacteria.

**Safety information:** Do not use horehound during pregnancy.

**Dosage advice:** Take 1–2 ml tincture mixed with 4 ounces of water or juice three or four times daily.

## Wild Cherry *(Prunus serotina)*

**Main actions:** Antitussive, sedative
**Part used:** Bark

Wild cherry bark is a well-known traditional remedy for coughs and is included in many herbal cough syrup formulas. Wild cherry bark helps calm the nerves that supply the bronchial passageways. This can alleviate the episodes of excessive and spasmodic coughing that often occur with COPD. However, do not use wild cherry when the cough is productive (brings up mucus), as this type of cough helps to clear the bronchial passageways of mucus.

**Safety information:** Wild cherry bark is generally considered safe when used as recommended.

**Dosage advice:** Take $^1/_2$–1 ml mixed tincture with 4 ounces of water two or three times daily.

## Yerba Santa *(Eriodictyon californicum)*

**Main action:** Expectorant
**Part used:** Leaf

Yerba santa is particularly useful for chronic bronchitis. It acts as an expectorant to help clear the bronchial passages of phlegm. It can be particularly useful in this manner when combined with grindelia (gumweed).

**Safety information:** Yerba santa is generally considered safe when used as directed.

**Dosage advice:** Take 1 ml mixed with 4 ounces of water two or three times daily.

## COMBINATION FORMULAS FOR COPD

Herbal infusions (teas) have a long history of use in medicine. Herbal teas not only provide you with a direct medicinal benefit, but they are also quite enjoyable, and they will serve as an excellent substitute for coffee or black tea. The formulas that follow are combinations of herbs to be prepared as an infusion and then drunk as a tea. Table 9 (see pages 144–145) gives a summary of all the herbs used in these formulas. It details the parts of the herb that should be used as well as the principal actions they provide.

The formulas begin on page 146 and they are organized into three groups: soothing formulas, expectorant formulas, and calming formulas. You may want to obtain the herbs in bulk, prepare the formulas according to the ratios given, and then store each dry formula in a labeled mason jar so that they are ready for use. Because the amount of each ingredient is given as a "part" (a unit of measurement that is up to you, as long as each part is equal), these recipes allow you to mix as much or as little of a formula as you want. If stored in a cool, dry area, the dry formulas will keep for several years.

Many of these herbs can be purchased in bulk at your local health food store. For mail-order sources of bulk herbs, see appendix 1.

## TABLE 9. HERBS USED IN COPD TEA FORMULAS

| Common Name | Botanical Name | Part(s) Used | Main Actions |
| --- | --- | --- | --- |
| Anise | *Pimpinella anisum* | Seed | Flavoring, antimicrobial, expectorant |
| Chamomile | *Matricaria recutita* | Flower | Antispasmodic, sedative |
| Elder | *Sambucus nigra* | Flower | Antimicrobial, anti-inflammatory, antiviral, immunomodulator |
| Elecampane | *Inula helenium* | Root | Antiseptic, expectorant |
| Fennel | *Foeniculum vulgare* | Seed | Antiseptic, mucolytic |
| Flax | *Linum usitatissimum* | Seed | Anti-inflammatory, demulcent |
| Horsetail | *Equisetum arvense* | Stem | Diuretic, astringent |
| Lavender | *Lavandula angustifolium* | Flower | Sedative |
| Licorice | *Glycyrrhiza glabra* | Root | Anti-inflammatory, expectorant, demulcent |
| Lungwort | *Pulmonaria officinalis* | Leaf | Demulcent, expectorant |
| Marshmallow | *Althaea officinalis* | Leaf, Root | Demulcent |

| Common Name | Botanical Name | Part(s) Used | Main Actions |
|---|---|---|---|
| Mullein | *Verbascum thapsus* | Leaf | Demulcent, expectorant, respiratory tonic |
| Nettle | *Urtica dioica* | Leaf | Immunomodulator, anti-inflammatory, tonic |
| Peppermint | *Mentha x piperata* | Leaf | Antispasmodic, tonic |
| Plantain | *Plantago* spp. | Leaf | Antibacterial, antimicrobial, anti-inflammatory, demulcent, expectorant |
| Sage | *Salvia officinalis* | Leaf | Antimicrobial, antispasmodic, astringent, antithrombotic |
| Thyme | *Thymus vulgaris* | Leaf | Antimicrobial, antiseptic |
| Valerian | *Valeriana officinalis* | Root | Antispasmodic, sedative |
| Wild cherry | *Prunus serotina* | Bark | Antitussive, sedative for the respiratory nerves |
| Yarrow | *Achillea millefolium* | Flower, leaf | Anti-inflammatory, astringent, tonic |

*Note:* Elecampane, flax, fennel, licorice root, sage, valerian, and yarrow should not be used during pregnancy.

### Soothing Formulas

The following formulas soothe bronchial passageways and help to heal damaged lung tissue.

**FORMULA 1**

| | |
|---|---|
| Flaxseed | 2 parts |
| Licorice root | 1 part |
| Marshmallow root | 1 part |

Infuse 1 teaspoon of formula in 1 cup of boiling water. Sweeten with honey if necessary. Use up to three times daily.

**FORMULA 2**

| | |
|---|---|
| Anise seed | 1 part |
| Fennel seed | 1 part |
| Licorice root | 1 part |
| Plantain leaves | 1 part |

Infuse 1 teaspoon of formula in 1 cup of boiling water. Sweeten with honey if necessary. Use up to three times daily.

**FORMULA 3**

| | |
|---|---|
| Licorice root | 1 part |
| Marshmallow leaf | 1 part |
| Marshmallow root | 1 part |
| Mullein | 1 part |

Infuse 1 teaspoon of formula in 1 cup of boiling water. Sweeten with honey if necessary. Use up to four times daily.

**FORMULA 4**

| | |
|---|---|
| Elecampane root | 1 part |
| Lungwort | 1 part |
| Nettle leaf | 1 part |
| Thyme | 1 part |

Infuse 1 teaspoon of formula in 1 cup of boiling water. Sweeten with honey if necessary. Use up to four times daily.

### *Expectorant Formulas*

These formulations help contain congestion, cough, and respiratory inflammation.

#### FORMULA 5

| | |
|---|---|
| Lungwort | 1 part |
| Mullein | 1 part |
| Plantain leaves | 1 part |

Infuse 1 teaspoon of formula in 1 cup of boiling water. Sweeten with honey if necessary. Use once daily.

#### FORMULA 6

| | |
|---|---|
| Plantain leaves | 4 parts |
| Lungwort | 2 parts |
| Nettle leaves | 2 parts |
| Yarrow flowers | 1 part |

Infuse 2 teaspoons of formula in 1 cup of boiling water. Sweeten with honey if necessary. Use once daily.

#### FORMULA 7

| | |
|---|---|
| Lungwort | 2 parts |
| Plantain leaves | 2 parts |
| Horsetail | 1 part |
| Nettle leaves | 1 part |

Infuse 3 teaspoons of formula in 1 cup of boiling water. Sweeten with honey if necessary. Use once daily.

#### FORMULA 8

| | |
|---|---|
| Yarrow flowers | 4 parts |
| Lungwort | 2 parts |
| Plantain leaf | 2 parts |
| Marshmallow root | 1 part |
| Sage | 1 part |

Infuse 1 teaspoon of formula in 1 cup of boiling water. Sweeten with honey if necessary. Use up to twice daily.

## FORMULA 9

| | |
|---|---|
| Elder flower | 4 parts |
| Elecampane root | 4 parts |
| Mullein | 4 parts |
| Thyme | 4 parts |
| Wild cherry bark | 4 parts |
| Peppermint leaf | 1 part |
| Sage | 1 part |

Infuse 3 teaspoons of formula in 1 cup of boiling water. Sweeten with honey if necessary. Use up to three times daily.

### Calming Formula

This formulation has a calming effect and can be used as a sedative.

## FORMULA 10

| | |
|---|---|
| Fennel seed | 3 parts |
| Yarrow flowers | 3 parts |
| Valerian root | 2 parts |
| Chamomile flowers | 1 part |
| Lavender flowers | 1 part |
| Peppermint leaf | 1 part |

Infuse 1 teaspoon of formula in 1 cup of boiling water. Use once daily.

### Other Herbs to Consider

The herbs in table 10 may also prove to be useful to varying degrees in addressing the issues related to your COPD.

Herbs, like other dietary supplements, work best when given an optimal environment in which to exert their effects. In other words, they are most effective when used in concert with dietary change and other natural health methods. Used as part of a holistic treatment plan, herbs can be remarkably effective in helping the body in its quest to heal itself.

## TABLE 10. OTHER HERBS TO CONSIDER FOR COPD

| Herb | Actions | Preparation |
|------|---------|-------------|
| Bilberry | Anti-inflammatory, antimicrobial | Take as a tea |
| Cat's claw | Antioxidant, anti-inflammatory, antiviral, immune system stimulant | Take as a liquid extract |
| Eucalyptus leaf and essential oil | Expectorant, anti-inflammatory, antibacterial | Take as a tea when using leaf; take by steam inhalation when using essential oil |
| Fenugreek | Expectorant | Take as a tea |
| Lobelia | Expectorant, relief of bronchial spasms | Take as a liquid extract |
| Red clover | Expectorant, antispasmodic | Take as a liquid extract |
| Slippery elm | Expectorant, protects mucous membranes | Take as a tea |

*Note:* Cat's claw, fenugreek, and lobelia are not to be used during pregnancy.

# 8

# Exercise, Breathing Techniques, and Other Physical Therapies

The primary aim of physical therapeutics for COPD is to improve breathing, restore one's ability to function in daily life, increase vitality, and improve quality of life. Exercise and physical therapeutics consist of activities such as walking and other aerobic exercise, special breathing techniques, yoga, qigong, t'ai chi, and massage therapy.

Physical activity is an essential part of maintaining health in general, and when it comes to building up the health of an individual with COPD, exercise and physical therapies should always be performed to the extent that this person can tolerate. The sedentary lifestyle that often accompanies COPD will ultimately contribute to a deterioration in functional capacity, cardiovascular function, and skeletal muscle mass. In order to avoid further health complications that can result from lack of activity, it is essential for you to maintain aerobic fitness and strength to the extent that you are able.

Exercise and physical therapeutics do not reverse damage related to COPD. However, exercise enables your muscles to adapt so they can extract oxygen from the blood more efficiently. Once that adaptation has occurred, you will experience less shortness of breath when you exert yourself.

Unlike therapeutic protocols such as diet and nutrition, nutritional supplements, and herbs, the degree to which COPD patients can become involved with exercise or physical therapies will always depend upon the status of their condition. Many COPD patients are elderly, and perhaps fragile or debilitated, and these are factors that will limit how much and what kind of exercise they can do. It is very important to consult your doctor before beginning any exercise program.

Yoga, qigong, and t'ai chi are forms of gentle exercise commonly performed in a group setting with the guidance of an experienced instructor. Once you learn the techniques, however, you can perform these activities at home.

## BREATHING TECHNIQUES

Two special breathing techniques especially helpful for people with COPD are pursed-lip breathing and diaphragmatic breathing. Pursed-lip breathing is a good method for helping to control dyspnea (shortness of breath). Diaphragmatic breathing helps improve the ability of the lungs to expand.

### Pursed-lip Breathing

Pursed-lip breathing is one of the easiest ways to control episodes of breathlessness. This technique is a quick and easy way to slow down your pace of breathing to make each breath more effective. Pursed-lip breathing helps to prolong exhalation, which then helps to slow down your breathing rate. Pursed-lip breathing also helps to improve ventilation of the lungs, keeps the airways open longer, and decreases the amount of work required for breathing. All of these factors contribute to easing your shortness of breath and helping you relax.

Perform pursed-lip breathing as follows: While relaxing your shoulders and your neck, inhale (take a normal breath) slowly through your nose while keeping your mouth closed. Then purse your lips—position them as you would if you were going to whistle. Slowly and gently exhale through your pursed lips. After you learn this technique, with a little practice you may utilize this technique whenever you find yourself having shortness of breath. Always make sure that your exhalation phase (breathing out) is longer than your inhalation phase (breathing in). If you are using pursed-lip breathing while engaged in an activity, always make sure you exhale during the strenuous part of the activity.

### Diaphragmatic Breathing

Diaphragmatic breathing helps your lungs expand so that they take in more air. This breathing technique will help to strengthen your diaphragm as well as help to decrease the work of breathing by slowing it down. When you practice this breathing technique, keep your chest, shoulders, and neck as relaxed as possible. The aim is to keep your upper body still and rely solely on your diaphragm.

Diaphragmatic breathing is performed as follows: Lie on your back on a flat surface, such as the floor or your bed, with a pillow under your knees and one under your head. Your knees should be slightly bent. Place your left hand on your upper chest and your right hand on your abdomen. This will enable you to feel your diaphragm move as you breathe. With your hands in place as just described, inhale slowly through your nose so that your stomach moves out against your right hand. You should be able to feel your right hand on your abdomen moving out. Your left hand on your chest should not move at all. Then tighten your stomach muscles and let them move back in as you exhale with the pursed-lip technique. As you are exhaling, you should be able to feel your right hand on your abdomen moving in, and your left hand on your chest should still not be moving at all. When you have perfected diaphragmatic breathing lying down, you can then do it while relaxing in a chair or even while standing. Diaphragmatic breathing should be practiced for five to ten minutes, three or four times a day.

Bending forward at the waist while breathing can also make it easier for you to breathe. As bending allows the diaphragm to move more easily, bending forward while breathing can decrease shortness of breath, even with individuals who have severe COPD. You may bend forward while doing pursed-lip breathing or diaphragmatic breathing if you are sitting or standing.

## WALKING AND OTHER AEROBIC EXERCISE

Aerobic exercise is physical activity that makes the heart and lungs work harder to meet the body's increased need for oxygen. Aerobic exercise also enhances the circulation of oxygen through the blood. In general, this kind of exercise increases your heart and breathing rate. Walking, jogging, swimming, dancing, cycling, and many other forms of exercise are all classified as aerobic because they increase the body's demand for oxygen.

Aerobic exercise can be extremely helpful for someone with COPD because it improves circulation and lung function as well as increasing stamina and building activity tolerance. Your ability to engage in aerobic exercise will depend on the severity of your condition and your general level of physical fitness. However, even someone with severe COPD can benefit from gentle aerobic exercise, such as walking. Again, be sure to consult your doctor before beginning any kind of exercise program.

Daily walking is one of the best exercise activities for a person with COPD. Walking will help your circulation and increase your stamina, and it will help build activity tolerance. Start out by walking half a block or less. Every other day, you should increase your walking distance a little bit. After a few months, you could be walking up to a mile without gasping for air. While you are walking, you should inhale through your nose and exhale through your mouth using the pursed-lip breathing technique.

Other forms of aerobic exercise appropriate for people with COPD are treadmill walking, bicycling or stationary cycling, and swimming. As many daily activities also require the use of the arms and the upper body, try to include endurance and strength training for your upper body in your exercise program. Consult with your physician or physical therapist to find out what types of endurance or strength training are most appropriate for your situation.

## YOGA

Yoga, one of the oldest health practices in the world, gets my highest endorsement as a physical therapy for people with COPD. Yoga is part of ayurveda, the traditional holistic health system of India, and has been practiced for thousands of years for its health benefits.

Yoga offers some of the best postural and breathing exercises in existence. The postures (asanas) provide excellent ways to gently develop strength and flexibility. Perhaps even more important in yoga are the breath-control techniques (pranayama), which can help a person with COPD breathe more easily and develop tolerance to more strenuous exercise. Yoga also promotes relaxation and can help reduce COPD-related emotional stress.

Individuals with COPD may find it helpful to begin practicing yoga with breath-control exercises to help strengthen the respiratory muscles. This can help you gain more control over breathlessness and increase your readiness for the physical postures of yoga as well as other forms of exercise. Even people with advanced COPD can benefit from simple yoga techniques.

The best way to get started with yoga is to take a class or work one-on-one with a trained yoga instructor. Many community recreation centers offer beginning yoga classes for people with physical disabilities. You can get more information on yoga and how to find a yoga instructor through the International Association of Yoga Therapists. You will find contact information for this organization in appendix 1.

## QIGONG AND T'AI CHI

Qigong and t'ai chi are gentle exercise practices that are part of the ancient holistic medicine system of China, known as traditional Chinese medicine, or TCM. Both qigong and t'ai chi combine slow, controlled physical movement with breath control to promote strength, balance, flexibility, relaxation, and overall well-being.

For people with COPD, the effects of practicing qigong or t'ai chi are similar to those of yoga. The physical exercises and breath-control techniques will help reduce breathlessness and lead to an overall increase in exercise tolerance. Qigong and t'ai chi also help improve balance, enhance circulation, and may even stimulate immune function.

Many community recreation centers and senior centers offer beginning t'ai chi classes. The following Web site has links for both t'ai chi and qigong: www.mtsu.edu/~jpurcell/Taichi/tc-links.htm.

## MASSAGE THERAPY

Massage therapy can be very helpful for people with respiratory disease. Massage therapy techniques helpful for COPD include postural drainage, manipulation of respiratory muscles combined with chest percussion, soft-tissue manipulation and joint mobilizations, and breathing exercises. When used as an adjunct therapy for COPD, massage therapy can help decrease shortness of breath, strengthen the muscles of respiration, improve forced vital capacity, reduce heart rate, increase oxygen saturation in the blood, and improve overall pulmonary functioning.

Massage therapy can also help with other problems caused by COPD such as decreased rib cage mobility and neck problems. Because COPD patients often utilize the accessory muscles of respiration in their neck in order to get oxygen to the lungs, these muscles in the neck become overtaxed as they work to compensate for the lack of normal movement in the rib cage.

Although massage therapy has specific therapeutic benefits for COPD, because it is also applied for the purpose of positively affecting your overall health and wel-being, it can be regarded as a natural holistic complement for both your general health and for the issues of your COPD. For more information on massage therapy as well as finding a practitioner, contact the American Massage Therapy Association. Its contact information is in appendix 1.

Exercise and physical therapeutics should be an integral component of your healing process. They can play an important role in helping you to improve your breathing, increase your functionality and vitality, and improve your quality of life.

# 9

# Other Alternatives and Considerations

In today's climate of increased awareness of natural health care options, people realize that the health care choices available to them reach far beyond the borders of conventional medicine. A flood of information is now available through books, the Internet, and the media. Given the vast amount of information on health and healing out there, people sometimes become bewildered by the number of choices they have. Making sense of all this information is one good reason to turn to a natural health practitioner for help.

Another good reason to seek the help of a qualified natural health practitioner is that some systems of medicine are inappropriate for use as self-treatment. Acupuncture, chiropractic, and homeopathy, for example, require the services of a practitioner specifically trained in the use of the therapies. This chapter provides a brief look at some of these systems of healing, as well as a discussion of environmental factors that can play an important role in helping you live with COPD.

## ACUPUNCTURE AND TRADITIONAL CHINESE MEDICINE

Traditional Chinese medicine is the ancient health system of China. This holistic system of medicine has developed over thousands of years and is still widely used both in China and around the world. Acupuncture—a treatment that involves the insertion of tiny needles into the skin to stimulate specific points on the body—has been an essential part of traditional Chinese medicine for more than five thousand years. Acupuncture has become more widely recognized and used in the United States and elsewhere as scientific research has confirmed many of its benefits. In addition to acupuncture, traditional Chinese medicine has its own complete system of herbal medicine.

Clinical evidence shows that acupuncture can be helpful for people with COPD. In studies, acupuncture has been shown to reduce shortness of breath, enhance ability to walk, and improve the results of pulmonary function testing (including $FEV_1$, RV, and TLC). The use of acupuncture in COPD can also help bring about a significant overall improvement in a person's quality of life.

I encourage you to consider acupuncture and traditional Chinese herbal medicine as part of your treatment plan for COPD. These therapies will complement any other natural therapeutic protocols you are using. Traditional Chinese medicine and acupuncture are based upon the principle that vital energy in the body (called *chi* or *qi*) flows along a series of channels known as meridians, which run throughout the body. When an individual is healthy, energy flows in a balanced manner along these meridians or channels. According to this philosophy, when a person has a disease, the energy flow along the meridians has become blocked or disrupted. Acupuncture involves inserting very fine needles into the skin at specific points that lie along these meridians to help rebalance the flow of chi and thereby promote health.

When performed by a licensed acupuncturist, acupuncture is quite safe. Some people may occasionally feel a slight sensation of pain at the needle site, but when done correctly, acupuncture usually does not hurt at all. The use of sterile, prepackaged, disposable acupuncture needles virtually eliminates any risk of infection.

Appendix 1 contains contact information for well-respected professional organizations that can provide you with additional information about acupuncture, traditional Chinese medicine, and how to find a licensed practitioner. Acufinder, in particular, has a very useful Web site that provides a great deal of general information about acupuncture as well as an extensive list of licensed practitioners.

## CHIROPRACTIC

Chiropractic is a system of health that revolves around the physical manipulation of the body to improve structural alignment. The philosophy behind the therapy is that misalignment of the spine (subluxation) can contribute to disease, because every cell, tissue, and organ in the body is ultimately connected to the nerves that run through the spinal column. While chiropractic is most often used to address pain, particularly back and neck pain, the fact is that chiropractic can play a vital role in a holistic treatment plan for COPD and myriad other health concerns.

According to chiropractic philosophy, misalignment of the spine interferes with the flow of nerve traffic in the body. This contributes to many health problems, such as back pain, respiratory and stomach disorders, and impaired immune system function. COPD does not result from misalignment of the spine; however, correcting the alignment of the spine allows for the proper and unobstructed flow of nerve transmission not only to the lungs, but also to every other organ essential to health. This is why chiropractic can be such a valuable addition to a holistic treatment plan to enhance lung function, build immunity, and support the body's innate healing abilities.

Another specific reason for including chiropractic in a treatment plan for COPD has to do with the mechanics of breathing. Various muscular parts of the respiratory system, including the diaphragm, have direct attachments to the spinal column. Misalignment of the spinal column can affect the optimal functioning of muscles essential for proper breathing, especially the diaphragm and the scalene muscles, both of which are directly attached to the spinal column.

Furthermore, as a consequence of COPD, air can become trapped in the lungs and push down on the diaphragm. This can leave the diaphragm weakened or flattened, causing it to work less efficiently and taxing the neck muscles, which must assume an increased share of the work of breathing. By maintaining the spinal column in its proper position, chiropractic can help the muscles essential to respiration to function optimally. In this respect, chiropractic can be especially beneficial for severe COPD.

Many chiropractors are trained in specific techniques to improve breathing and enhance overall health. See appendix 1 for contact information for professional organizations that can help you find a licensed chiropractor in your area.

## ENVIRONMENTAL FACTORS

Exercising awareness of your environment can play a significant role in reducing or eliminating potential irritation to your lungs. People with COPD also need to stay aware of and minimize factors in their environment that can contribute to an increased risk of infections. Here are some guidelines for limiting the irritants in your environment.

1. Keep your home as clean and free of dust and mold as possible, especially your bedroom and bathroom. At minimum, a third of your life is spent in your bedroom, so be extra conscious about this room.
2. Keep your nebulizer clean and change the tubing often. If you have a suction catheter, keep the container clean and change the tubing often. If you use direct aerosol humidification, keep the machine and the cup clean and change the tubing often. Clean your nebulizer by washing it in warm soapy water with a clean cloth, then rinse thoroughly and allow to air dry. You may also wipe it with an alcohol wipe.
3. Do not use handkerchiefs or cloth towels to take care of mucus— use tissues or paper towels and dispose of them immediately.
4. Reduce clutter as much as possible. This effectively reduces the surface area on which dust and germs can collect.
5. Empty trashcans as frequently as possible.

6. Use air-cleaning machines, both circulating and electrostatic, throughout your home, especially in your bedroom, and change the filters regularly. Electrostatic air-cleaning machines are ideal for removing small particles from the air, while circulating air-cleaning machines remove larger particles; using the two together will provide the broadest, most thorough cleansing. Depending upon how much money you want to spend, you can get freestanding portable units or you can have an air purification system installed in the the duct system of your home. Reasonably priced, good-quality air filtration units are available at discount and home improvement stores. Just be sure whatever unit you buy has a HEPA (high efficiency particulate air) filter as a component part of the machine.

7. Air conditioning, especially filtered central air conditioning, is beneficial for people with COPD. If you live in a hot and humid climate, it is essential.

8. Use a humidifier as much as possible, and be sure to clean the machine frequently to prevent bacterial growth. Humidification is essential for individuals who have thick and copious mucus secretions. It helps to loosen the secretions and it makes them easier to expectorate.

9. Be sure the flooring in your home is hardwood, ceramic tile, or stone. Carpets retain dirt, dust, chemicals, mold, and many other irritants that are detrimental to COPD.

10. Use wood or plastic blinds as window coverings in your home. Drapes and curtains also retain dirt and dust that are irritating to your lungs.

11. The hair and dander of furry or feathered animals are deleterious to your condition.

12. Avoid anything that is potentially irritating to the lungs, including perfumes, colognes, scented laundry products, aerosol products, cleaners, solvents, paint, glue, and other inhaled chemical substances.

13. Avoid inhaling any gas or fumes from a gas stove. If you use a gas stove, consider replacing it with an electric stove.

14. Do not smoke, and never allow anyone to smoke in your home or car.
15. Avoid any and all dirty, dusty, moldy, or otherwise toxic environments.
16. Avoid stressful situations.
17. Get plenty of rest and fresh air.

## HOMEOPATHY

Homeopathy is a system of medicine that is probably very different from others with which you might be familiar. Homeopathy may be best described as "energetic medicine" in the sense that its medicinal effects do not follow the laws of chemistry the way those of drugs and herbs do. While scientists have not yet pinpointed how homeopathy works, this system of medicine has enjoyed safe and effective clinical use for more than two hundred years.

Homeopathic remedies are highly diluted and contain no more than trace amounts of active ingredients. The ingredients upon which homeopathic remedies are based may come from plants, minerals, animals, and many other sources. You may be wondering how a remedy can have a medicinal effect if no molecules of the active ingredient remain in the remedy. The answer lies in the realm of physics, not chemistry. Drugs and herbs work in ways that involve chemistry (in other words, physical interactions between molecules and cells). Homeopathic remedies, however, work on a whole different plane. The energetic principles that govern the way these remedies work are the subject of ongoing research.

If you want to use homeopathy successfully in your efforts to minimize your COPD symptoms and rebuild your health, you must work with a well-trained, skilled homeopathic practitioner (also known as a homeopath). You cannot expect to have any real success if you attempt to use homeopathy on your own, for self-treatment. This is not because homeopathy is not safe; it's because only a skilled practitioner will be able to find the remedy that is most appropriate for you and your specific symptoms.

For example, your main complaints may be excessive mucus and shortness of breath. The homeopathic practitioner, however, may ask you about your sleep habits, whether you prefer hot or cold beverages, whether your congestion is worse at night or in the morning, or whether you feel better outside in the fresh air or indoors. These are but a few of the many questions a homeopath might ask in order to establish a complete picture of your overall health status and your COPD in order to determine the best treatment.

Homeopathy cannot cure emphysema or COPD. However, when the appropriate remedy is selected, homeopathy can play a significant role in reducing inflammation and shortness of breath, strengthening immunity, increasing vitality, and improving overall health. Appendix 1 contains information on how to find a qualified and skilled homeopathic practitioner.

In closing, I want to wish you well and offer you encouragement as you begin the process to build back your health. This book is just the beginning for you. The wisdom of natural medicine is timeless and is based upon principles that have served humankind throughout the ages. Learn it well and allow it to serve you in your quest to heal. My prayers are always with you.

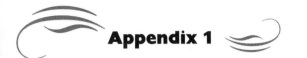

## Appendix 1

# Additional Resources

The organizations listed in this appendix can help you find a natural health care practitioner, purchase products you need, and obtain more information.

## FINDING A HEALTH CARE PRACTITIONER

These organizations generally have good reputations, but always use your own discretion to determine the suitability of any particular organization, company, or practitioner to serve your needs.

### Acupuncture and Oriental Medicine

**Acufinder**
825 College Boulevard, Suite 102–211
Oceanside, CA 92057
760-630-3600
www.acufinder.com

**Acupuncture and Oriental Medicine Alliance**
PO Box 378
Gig Harbor, WA 98335
253-238-8134
www.www.aomalliance.org

**American Association of Oriental Medicine**
PO Box 162340
Sacramento, CA 95816
916-443-4770
www.aaom.org

## Chiropractors

**National Directory of Chiropractic Foundation**
406 E 300 South, Box 305
Salt Lake City, UT 84111
800-888-7914
www.chirodirectory.com

## Holistic Physicians (MD and DO)

**American Holistic Medical Association**
PO Box 2016
Edmonds, WA 98020
425-967-0737
www.holisticmedicine.org

**American College for Advancement in Medicine**
24411 Ridge Route, Suite 115
Laguna Hills, CA 92653
949-309-3520
www.acamnet.org

## Herbalists and Herb Information

**American Herbalists Guild**
141 Nob Hill Road
Cheshire, CT 06410
203-272-6731
www.americanherbalistsguild.com

**American Botanical Council**
6200 Manor Road
Austin, TX 78723
512-926-4900
www.herbalgram.org

## Homeopathic Practitioners

**National Center for Homeopathy**
801 N. Fairfax Street, Suite 306
Alexandria, VA 22314
703-548-7790
877-624-0613
www.homeopathic.org

**North American Society of Homeopaths**
PO Box 450039
Sunrise, FL 33345
206-720-7000
www.homeopathy.org

## Hypnotherapists

**National Guild of Hypnotists**
PO Box 308
Merrimack, NH 03054
603-429-9438
www.ngh.net

## Naturopaths and Other Natural Health Practitioners

### American Association of Naturopathic Physicians
4435 Wisconsin Avenue NW, Suite 403
Washington, DC 20016
866-538-2267
www.naturopathic.org

### National Association of Certified Natural Health Professionals
710 East Winona Avenue
Warsaw, IN 46580
800-321-1005
www.cnhp.org

### American Holistic Health Association
PO Box 17400
Anaheim, CA 92817
714-779-6152
www.ahha.org

## Nutrition Professionals

### American Association of Nutritional Consultants
401 Kings Highway
Winona Lake, IN 46590
888-828-2262
www.aanc.net

### National Association of Nutrition Professionals
PO Box 1172
Danville, CA 94526
800-342-8037
www.nanp.org

## Orthomolecular Medicine

**International Society for Orthomolecular Medicine**
16 Florence Avenue
Toronto, Ontario
Canada M2N 1E9
416-733-2117
www.orthomed.org

## SOURCES FOR PRODUCTS

The following companies are those I have had experience with in purchasing nebulizers, compounded medications, and dietary supplements, including bulk herbs.

## Nebulizer Equipment

From my own experience I recommend MisterNeb, Respironics, and Omron as affordable, quality nebulizer brands. Allergy Be Gone is a reputable company in New York that carries all of these brands, and people there are available to answer questions you may have as well as provide information on the use, care, and cleaning of a nebulizer.

**Allergy Be Gone**
140 58th Street, Suite 7K
Brooklyn, NY 11220
866-234-6630
www.allergybegone.com

## Nebulizer Glutathione

Medaus Pharmacy, a compounding pharmacy in Birmingham, Alabama, is well versed in making nebulizer-grade reduced glutathione. The company has indicated that it may be able to prepare and ship the COPD Nebulizer Formula described in chapter 6.

Medaus has a referral network of physicians all over the United States that it works with regularly. If you call and say where you live, Medaus can refer you to the physician in its network who is closest to your area.

**Medaus Pharmacy & Compounding Center**
2637 Valleydale Road
Birmingham, AL 35244
800-526-9183
www.medaus.com

## Colloidal Silver

Mesosilver, made by Purest Colloids in New Jersey, is regarded as one of the best colloidal silver products on the market today, and is the only form of colloidal silver that I use. Mesosilver can be taken internally or via a nebulizer.

**Purest Colloids, Inc.**
600 Highland Drive, Suite 602
Westhampton, NJ 08060
866-233-4633
609-267-6284
www.purestcolloids.com

## Bulk Herbs

**Mountain Rose Herbs**
PO Box 50220
Eugene, OR 97405
800-879-3337
www.mountainroseherbs.com

## Herbal Extracts

**Nature's Answer**
75 Commerce Drive
Hauppauge, NY 11788
800-439-2324
www.naturesanswer.com

**Eclectic Institute, Inc.**
36350 SE Industrial Way
Sandy, OR 97055
800-332-4372
www.eclecticherb.com
www.eclecticwater.com

**Wise Woman Herbals, Inc.**
PO Box 279
Creswell, OR 97426
541-895-5172
www.wisewomanherbals.com

## Green Food Supplements

Greens for Life, by Formulations for Life, is an excellent green food supplement in powder form that is mixed with water or juice. In addition to its content of many green vegetables, Greens for Life contains milk thistle, bromelain, grape seed extract, quercetin, and probiotics, all of which are important for an individual with COPD.

**Formulations for Life**
31 Harbor Hills Drive
Port Washington, NY 11050
516-467-4322
www.formulationsforlife.com

## Juicers

Juicer prices and capabilities vary. For making wheatgrass juice, the Miracle MJ-550 is quite good; it costs around $150. For citrus, the Omega Citrus Juicer 5000 is a great choice at around $139. For about $100, the Juiceman Jr. Juicer will handle all the rest of your fruits and vegetables. If you are able to make a more substantial investment and get a juicer that will handle everything, the Samson Ultra Juicer, at $400, is the way to go.

## Vitamins and Minerals

I recommend purchasing vitamins and supplements from the following companies. In a day and age when countless companies are marketing nutritional supplements, you can be assured that those listed here conform to the highest standards of the industry and manufacture products of the highest quality.

**Food Science of Vermont**
20 New England Drive
Essex Junction, VT 05453
800-874-9444
www.foodsciencevt.com

**Integrative Therapeutics, Inc.**
Customer Service Department
825 Challenger Drive
Green Bay, WI 54311
800-931-1709
www.integrativeinc.com

**Natrol**
21411 Prairie Street
Chatsworth, CA 91311
818-739-6000
www.natrol.com

**Nordic Naturals, Inc. (fish oil)**
94 Hangar Way
Watsonville, CA 95076
800-662-2544
www.nordicnaturals.com

**Nutraceutical International Corp.**
1400 Kearns Boulevard, 2nd Floor
Park City, UT 84060
800-669-8877
www.nutraceutical.com

**Pure Encapsulations, Inc.**
490 Boston Post Road
Sudbury, MA 01776
800-753-2277
www.purecaps.com
*(Pure Encapsulation products are available only through health care practitioners.)*

**Seroyal USA**
827 N. Central Avenue
Wood Dale, IL 60191
888-737-6925
www.seroyal.com

**Solgar Vitamin and Herb**
500 Willow Tree Road
Leonia, NJ 07605
1-877-SOLGAR4
www.solgar.com

## OTHER PRACTITIONERS AND SERVICES

**International Association of Yoga Therapists**
115 S. McCormick Street, Suite 3
Prescott, AZ 86303
928-541-0004
www.iayt.org

**American Massage Therapy Association**
500 Davis Street, Suite 900
Evanston, IL 60201
888-843-2682
877-905-2700
www.amtamassage.org

**American Physical Therapy Association**
1111 N. Fairfax Street
Alexandria, VA 22314
800-999-2782
703-684-2782
www.apta.org

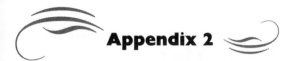

# Appendix 2

# Recommended Reading

## ACUPRESSURE

*Acupressure Techniques: Well-being and Pain Relief at Your Fingertips,* by Julian Kenyon, MD (Healing Arts Press)

Like acupuncture, acupressure involves the stimulation of specific points on the body. The difference is that instead of tiny needles, acupressure utilizes deep finger pressure over acupuncture points. In this fine book, Dr. Julian Kenyon presents a variety of acupressure techniques that are easy to learn and apply for a wide range of health conditions. It includes five specific points where pressure can be applied to help with the phlegm associated with bronchitis.

## BACH FLOWER REMEDIES

*Advanced Bach Flower Therapy: A Scientific Approach to Diagnosis and Treatment,* by Götz Blome, MD (Healing Arts Press)

Today even practitioners of conventional medicine recognize that there is often a distinct relationship between physical illness and a person's psychological or emotional condition. More than fifty years ago, Dr. Edward Bach discovered the use of flower essences for treating the mental and emotional aspects of illness. No matter what your physical illness, the application of Bach Flower remedies can help restore your psychological well-being and benefit your health overall, especially if you have a chronic condition.

## ENZYMES

*Enzymes: The Key to Health,* by Howard F. Loomis Jr., DC, FIACA (21st Century Nutrition Publishing)

Enzymes play an essential role in good health and disease prevention, and much of the food found in the typical American grocery is enzyme deficient. In this book, Dr. Loomis explains the importance of naturally occurring enzymes in whole foods for adequate digestion and assimilation of nutrients by the body. When enzymes are missing from food due to overprocessing, the digestive problems that result eventually give rise to myriad health problems. This book makes an excellent case for the need to adopt a whole foods diet in order to acquire the nutrients essential for building health and warding off disease.

## GENERAL HEALTH

*Fell's Official Know-It-All Guide to Health & Wellness,* by Dr. M. Ted Morter Jr. (Frederick Fell Publishers, Inc.)

This easy-to-use guide is a valuable reference on nutrition and its effects on human health. One of the main objectives of the book is help the reader understand the pH (acidity or alkalinity) of foods, which directly affects the body's acid–alkaline balance and consequently the health status of the individual. Dr. Morter establishes a sensible and scientifically valid approach to eating that optimizes the internal pH of the body.

## HERBS

*Herbal Prescriptions after 50* (new edition of *An Elders' Herbal*), by David Hoffmann (Healing Arts Press)

*Herbal Remedies for Dummies,* by Christopher Hobbs, LAc (For Dummies)

*The Herb Book,* by John B. Lust (Bantam Books)

*The New Holistic Herbal,* by David Hoffmann (Healing Arts Press)

*Nutritional Herbology,* by Mark Pedersen (Wendell W. Whitman)

*Planetary Herbology,* by Michael Tierra, ND, OMD (Lotus Press)

David Hoffmann, Christopher Hobbs, and Michael Tierra are among the most respected medical herbalists in the world today. Their books present a holistic approach to herbal medicine that will help readers build a foundation from which to begin using herbs to promote health. Dr. Tierra's *Planetary Herbology* is his classic treatise integrating Western herbalism with the traditional Chinese and Indian systems of herbal medicine.

Mark Pedersen's *Nutritional Herbology* is one of the few books I have seen in which a complete nutritional profile (content of vitamins, minerals, carbohydrates, proteins, etc.) is given for many commonly used herbs. *The Herb Book,* by the renowned American naturopath John B. Lust, is a classic paperback compendium of essentially every American herb known. Although many advances have been made in our knowledge of herbs in the years since its publication in 1974, it is still a great way to introduce yourself to the world of herbs.

## HERBAL MEDICINE MAKING

The books listed here provide clear, concise, and practical information on the preparation and use of traditional herbal medicines.

*The Herbal Medicine Cabinet,* by Debra St. Claire (Celestial Arts)

*Handmade Medicines: Simple Recipes for Herbal Health,* by Christopher Hobbs, LAc (Interweave Press)

*From the Shepherd's Purse,* by Max G. Barlow (Spice West Publications); available through www.reagansbookstore.com

In my opinion, this is a must-have book for anyone involved in making his or her own medicinal herb preparations. It includes a discussion of plant structure and identification, and gives instruction on the collection, drying, and storage of botanicals. The hallmark of this book, though, is its detailed descriptions of how to prepare tinctures and fluid extracts, infusions and decoctions, and poultices, ointments, and salves.

## JUICING

*Juicing for Life,* by Cherie Calbom (Avery Publishing)

In *Juicing for Life,* Cherie Calbom provides a safe, effective, and natural way to achieve better health through juicing. She explains the various fruits and vegetables that have been found to be effective against certain diseases as well as giving specific juicing information for more than seventy-five different health conditions. Also included in the book are numerous juicing recipes as well as several diet plans to use in conjunction with your juicing program.

*Juiceman's Power of Juicing,* by Jay Kordich (Morrow Cookbooks)

As one of the original pioneers of the juicing movement, Jay Kordich has been advocating the nutritional value of juicing for over fifteen years. Kordich explores the nutritional values of assorted fruits and vegetables, and offers useful information about purchasing and storing perishable produce. The book is filled with delicious recipes that will enhance your juicing experience.

*The Juicing Bible,* by Pat Crocker (Robert Rose)

Complete with charts and tables, this book discusses more than one hundred different fruits, vegetables, and herbs that may be used for juicing. Replete with juicing recipes, this book also discusses smoothies and medicinal teas. There are many unusual recipes that will stretch the boundaries and broaden the horizons of the juicing experience.

## NUTRITION

*Diet & Nutrition: A Holistic Approach,* by Rudolph Ballentine, MD (Himalayan Institute Press)

At 634 pages, Dr. Ballentine's *Diet & Nutrition* is one of the most comprehensive texts on holistic nutrition to be found in a single volume. It is an outstanding introduction to holistic nutrition and lays a firm foundation for understanding the relationship between diet and health in all of its aspects. A hallmark of the book is Dr. Ballentine's skillful synthesis of the nutritional insights of Eastern medicine with the scientific research of the West.

*Encyclopedia of Healing Foods,* by Michael Murray, Joseph Pizzorno, and Lara Pizzorno (Atria Books)

This comprehensive and practical book is a guide to the nutritional benefits and medicinal qualities of just about every edible substance.

## ORTHOMOLECULAR MEDICINE

*Putting It All Together: The New Orthomolecular Nutrition,* by Abram Hoffer, MD, PhD, and Morton Walker, DPM (introduction by Linus Pauling, PhD) (Keats Publishing)

Orthomolecular medicine approaches disease through an understanding of individual biochemistry and seeks to correct illness by providing the body with optimal amounts of substances that are natural to it. This book, a revised and expanded edition of the classic *Orthomolecular Nutrition,* by pioneers Linus Pauling and Abram Hoffer, delivers a thorough overview of orthomolecular nutrition in easily understood language. The book discusses optimal diet, the three components of nutrition, and vitamin and mineral supplements, as well as strategies for overcoming illness and building optimal health.

## RAW FOODS

*Living Foods for Optimum Health: Staying Healthy in an Unhealthy World,* by Brian R. Clement (Prima Publishing)

*The Complete Book of Raw Food: Healthy, Delicious Vegetarian Cuisine Made with Living Foods,* edited by Lori Baird (Healthy Living Books)

*Living Cuisine: The Art and Spirit of Raw Foods,* by Renée Loux Underkoffler (Avery)

To help you get started incorporating raw foods into your diet, I recommend three great books. *Living Foods for Optimum Health* is the best place to start if you have no experience with eating a raw foods diet. The other two excellent books I've listed here are packed with recipes and tons of other information on eating raw foods.

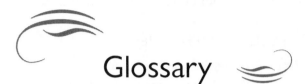

# Glossary

**acute.** Used to describe an illness that begins abruptly with marked intensity, but then subsides after a relatively short period of time.

**acinus.** The ending of the airway in the lungs where the alveoli (air sacs) are located; respiratory bronchioles and their alveolar sacs are collectively known as the acinus. The acinus is essentially a lobule without the terminal bronchiole, and it is where actual gas exchange in the lungs occurs. The acinus is something like a cluster of grapes, in which the main stem coming off the vine is the respiratory bronchiole, the smaller stems are the alveolar ducts, and the grapes themselves are the alveoli.

**alveoli.** The tiny air-containing sacs that are the endpoint of the respiratory passageways within the lungs. The alveoli are where the exchange of oxygen and carbon dioxide takes place.

**antioxidant.** A substance that works to prevent damage to the body's cells from unstable molecules called free radicals. The normal cellular processes of oxidation in our bodies produce highly reactive free radicals. Free radicals are also contained in cigarette smoke. COPD patients have significant amounts of oxidative damage in their lungs due to free radicals. Free radicals readily react with and damage other molecules and cells. Antioxidants are capable of "mopping up" free radicals before they damage other essential molecules or cells.

**antiprotease.** A protein that has the ability to inhibit the activity of a protease. Alpha-1 antitrypsin is an anti-protease that inhibits the activity of the protease neutrophil elastase.

**antitussive.** A substance that helps to relieve coughing.

**atypical.** Refers to a situation or condition that is different from what would be considered usual or typical.

**bronchiole.** A tiny tube in the respiratory passageways within the lung that is a continuation of the bronchi and connects to the alveoli (the air sacs).

**bronchoconstriction.** Narrowing of the bronchi or bronchioles.

**bronchodilation.** Widening of the bronchi or bronchioles.

**bronchodilator.** A substance that helps improve airflow through the lungs. Bronchodilators act by relaxing bronchial smooth muscle, allowing the respiratory passageways to expand and thus permitting greater airflow through the lungs.

**bulla** (bullae, plural). An enlarged airspace greater than 1 cm (a little less than a half inch) in diameter that can be present with any of the four types of emphysema. Bullae occupy areas right next to the visceral pleura, usually near the apex (top) of the lungs. When these localized areas are especially prominent, the condition is sometimes referred to as bullous emphysema.

**bullectomy.** The surgical removal of a bulla, which is a large, distended air space in the lung that does not contribute to breathing function. Once the bulla is removed, the healthy air sacs around it have room to expand, and the muscles used to breathe can function better.

**carminative.** A substance that helps to relieve gas in the stomach and the bowels.

**catalyst.** A substance that influences the rate of a chemical reaction without becoming consumed or permanently altered in the process.

**chemotactic.** The tendency of cells to migrate either toward or away from a chemical stimulus.

**chemotaxis.** A response that involves movement either toward or away from a chemical stimulus.

**chronic.** Describes a disease or disorder that develops slowly and persists over a long period of time.

**cilia.** Small, hairlike structures on the outer surfaces of some cells. Some of the respiratory epithelium contains cilia, which aid in the process of removing mucus and debris from the respiratory tract.

**collagen.** The main protein in connective tissue. Collagen is a long, fibrous structural protein that supports most tissues.

**connective tissue.** One of the fundamental tissue types found in the human body. There are several types of connective tissue, one of which is loose connective tissue, which holds organs and epithelia in place. Loose connective tissue contains a variety of fibers including collagen and elastin.

**contraindication.** Any factor that would prohibit the use of a drug, supplement, herb, or other therapeutic protocol.

**cytokine.** A small protein molecule that acts as a messenger between cells of the immune system, and between immune system cells and other cell types.

**cytoplasm.** Essentially, all the internal contents of a cell except for the nucleus. It is a jellylike material, consisting mainly of water, that contains all of the cell's organelles along with salts, organic molecules, and many enzymes.

**diaphoretic.** A substance that promotes perspiration.

**distal.** Away from or farthest from a point of origin.

**dysplasia.** Any abnormal cellular development or change, such as alteration in size, shape, or organization of cells, that occurs within tissues or organs.

**dyspnea.** Breathlessness, shortness of breath.

**edema.** Abnormal accumulation of fluid in the interstitial spaces of tissues. Interstitial spaces are the spaces between tissues.

**elastase.** Elastase is an enzyme from the class of proteases that break down proteins.

**elastin.** A protein that is the principal constituent of elastic tissue fibers. The elastic fibers found in the interalveolar septum (alveolar wall) are destroyed by the enzyme neutrophil elastase.

**enzyme.** A protein that is produced by living cells that acts as a catalyst for the chemical reactions that occur within the organism. Most enzymes catalyze reactions that occur within the cell that produces the enzyme.

**epithelium.** One of the four fundamental tissues of the human body. Epithelial tissue is composed of a layer of cells that can be found covering body surfaces; lining hollow organs, body cavities, and ducts; and forming glands. Epithelium includes the cells that line the inside of the respiratory tract.

**eosinophil.** A type of white blood cell responsible for fighting infection in the body.

**expectorant.** A substance that facilitates the removal of mucus and phlegm from the bronchial passageways.

**fibrosis.** Proliferation of fibrous connective tissue. The process of fibrosis is normal in the formation of scar tissue that replaces normal tissue lost through injury or infection; it can become abnormal when the fibrous connective tissue spreads over or replaces normal smooth muscle or other normal tissue.

**flavonoid.** A plant chemical that exerts a wide range of biological effects, including antioxidant and anti-inflammatory effects.

**gluten.** A protein found in wheat. It is a sticky, elastic substance formed when gliadin and glutenin, two insoluble proteins also found in wheat, are combined when wheat is moistened and kneaded.

**goblet cells.** Specialized cells that secrete mucus and form glands in the epithelium of the respiratory tract, stomach, and intestines.

**hemoglobin.** A complex, iron-containing protein molecule contained within red blood cells that enables them to bind and carry oxygen.

**histamine.** A protein that acts as a chemical transmitter in local immune responses, regulation of stomach acid production, and allergic reactions as a mediator of hypersensitivity. It causes an inflammatory response as well as contraction of smooth muscle, which induces bronchoconstriction.

**holistic.** In medical terms, an approach to health and living that considers the entirety of an individual's well-being. This includes addressing the physical, mental, and emotional aspects of an individual as well as promoting nutritional and lifestyle modifications that will lead to a healthy existence.

**hyperplasia.** An increase in the number of the cells of an organ or tissue that causes it to increase in size.

**hypertrophy.** An increase in the size of an organ or tissue that occurs due to an increase in cell size, rather than cell division.

**hypoxia.** A condition that occurs when there is a deficiency in the amount of oxygen reaching body tissues.

**hypoxemia.** Insufficient oxygenation of the blood.

**immunomodulator.** A substance that affects the function of the immune system, the body's built-in system of defense against disease. Immuno-modulators can be either immunostimulants or immunosuppresants.

**inhibitor.** A substance that prevents or restricts a certain action, such as the activity of an enzyme.

**leukocyte.** An umbrella term for white blood cells. Leukocytes are subdivided into lymphocytes, monocytes, neutrophils, basophils, and eosinophils.

**leukotriene.** A messenger molecule that is part of the family of molecules known as eicosanoids; leukotrienes play an important role in the inflammatory response.

**lipid peroxidation.** Oxidative deterioration of lipids as a result of oxidative stress. Lipid peroxidation is a free radical–related process that causes cellular damage.

**lymphocyte.** A type of white blood cell (leukocyte) that develops in the bone marrow and plays an integral part in the body's defenses. Lymphocytes occur as B cells, which are involved in antigen–antibody immune responses (humoral immunity), and T cells, which are involved in cell-mediated immunity.

**lobule.** A collective term for the terminal bronchioles along with their respective respiratory bronchioles and alveolar sacs.

**metaplasia.** The conversion of normal tissue cells into an abnormal form in response to chronic stress or injury. See *dysplasia*.

**mucolytic.** A substance that dissolves or destroys mucus.

**mucous membrane.** The thin layer of tissue that lines or covers the cavities or canals of the body that are open to the outside. Mucous membranes line the respiratory passages, the digestive tract, and the urogenital tract. Mucous membranes consist of a surface layer of epithelium that covers a deeper layer of connective tissue.

**nasopharynx.** The part of the pharynx that lies behind the nose and above the level of the soft palate.

**naturopath** (ND). An individual who has completed a curriculum of study and has been awarded the doctor of naturopathy (ND) degree. Traditional naturopaths are primarily teachers who educate clients on approaches to healthful living and building health through noninvasive natural means. True naturopathy never involves the use of drugs, surgery, or any invasive procedures.

**necrosis.** Localized tissue death that occurs in groups of cells in response to injury or disease.

**neutrophil elastase.** A protease that breaks down the protein elastin in the alveolar wall.

**nucleus.** The "command center" of the cell; an organelle that contains the genetic material necessary to maintain the functions of the cell.

**pathogenic.** Capable of causing or producing disease or illness.

**pH.** A measure of the relative acidity or alkalinity of a solution. pH is measured on a scale of 0–14 with 7 being neutral, less than 7 being acidic, and greater than 7 being alkaline or basic.

**polymorphonuclear.** Having a multilobed nucleus, such as a neutrophil. A neutrophil is a polymorphonuclear leukocyte.

**protease.** An enzyme that breaks down proteins. See *elastase*.

**reducing agent.** A substance that donates electrons to another substance in a chemical reaction.

**smooth muscle.** A type of muscle tissue that is not under voluntary control, found principally with the internal organs. Smooth muscle surrounds the bronchi and bronchioles of the respiratory tract.

**standardized extract.** A highly processed herb extract that contains a guaranteed amount of one or more chemical compounds.

**subepithelial.** Refers to the area beneath the epithelium.

**submucosal.** Refers to the layer of loose connective tissue beneath a mucous membrane.

**synergistic, synergy.** The process by which two or more substances work together simultaneously to enhance the function and effect of one another.

**therapeutic.** Something that has healing properties or is beneficial in healing.

**thoracic cavity.** The space enclosed by the ribs, sternum, and diaphragm, containing the heart, lungs, esophagus, and thymus gland.

**tonic.** A substance that helps to restore normal tone and function to the tissues of the body.

**vasoconstriction.** Narrowing of a blood vessel.

**vasodilation.** Widening of a blood vessel.

# Selected Bibliography

Alberts, Bruce, Alexander Johnson, Julian Lewis, Martin Raff, Keith Roberts, and Peter Walter. *Molecular Biology of the Cell.* 4th ed. New York: Garland Science, 2002.

Anderson, Kenneth N., Lois E. Anderson, and Walter D. Glanze, eds. *Mosby's Medical, Nursing, and Allied Health Dictionary.* 4th ed. St. Louis, MO: Mosby, 1994.

Balch, Phyllis A., and James F. Balch. *Prescription for Nutritional Healing.* 3rd ed. New York: Avery, 2000.

Bellavite, Paolo, and Andrea Signorini. *The Emerging Science of Homeopathy: Complexity, Biodynamics, and Nanopharmacology.* Berkeley, CA: North Atlantic Books, 2002.

Braunwald, Eugene, Anthony S. Fauci, Dennis L. Kasper, Stephen L. Hauser, Dan L. Longo, and J. Larry Jameson. *Harrison's Principles of Internal Medicine.* 15th ed. New York: McGraw-Hill, 2001.

Champe, Pamela C., Richard A. Harvey, and Denise R. Ferrier. *Lippincott's Illustrated Reviews: Biochemistry.* 3rd ed. Philadelphia: Lippincott, Williams & Wilkins, 2005.

Chandra, V., Jayasankar Jasti, Punit Kaur, Ch. Betzel, A. Srinivasan, and T. P. Singh. "First Structural Evidence of a Specific Inhibition of Phospholipase $A_2$ by $\alpha$-tocopherol (vitamin E) and Its Implications in Inflammation: Crystal Structure of the Complex Formed Between Phospholipase $A_2$ and $\alpha$-tocopherol at 1.8 Å Resolution." *Journal of Molecular Biology* 320 (2002): 215–22.

185

Cooper, Geoffrey M. *The Cell: A Molecular Approach*. Sunderland, MA: Sinauer Associates, 1997.

Cotran, Ramzi S., Vinay Kumar, and Tucker Collins. *Robbins Pathologic Basis of Disease*. 6th ed. Philadelphia: W. B. Saunders, 1999.

Grippi, Michael A. *Pulmonary Pathophysiology*. Philadelphia: Lippincott, Williams & Wilkins, 1995.

Gruenwald, Joerg, Thomas Brendler, and Christof Jaenicke, eds. *PDR for Herbal Medicines*. 2nd ed. Montvale, NJ: Thomson Healthcare, 2000.

Guyton, Arthur C., and John E. Hall. *Textbook of Medical Physiology*. 10th ed. Philadelphia: W. B. Saunders, 2000.

Hendler, Sheldon S., and David Rorvik, eds. *PDR for Nutritional Supplements*. Montvale, NJ: Thomson Healthcare, 2001.

Lust, John. *The Herb Book*. New York: Bantam Books, 1974.

Lust, John, and Michael Tierra. *The Natural Remedy Bible*. New York: Pocket Books, 1990.

Murray, Michael, and Joseph Pizzorno. *Encyclopedia of Natural Medicine*. 2nd ed. Rocklin, CA: Prima Health, 1998.

Netter, Frank H. *Atlas of Human Anatomy*. 2nd ed. East Hanover, NJ: Novartis, 1997.

Pedersen, Mark. *Nutritional Herbology*. Warsaw, IN: Wendell W. Whitman Company, 2002.

Pentland, Alice P., Aubrey R. Morrison, Susan C. Jacobs, Luciann Lisi Hruza, Jason S. Hebert, and Lester Packer. "Tocopherol Analogs Suppress Arachidonic Acid Metabolism via Phospholipase Inhibition." *Journal of Biological Chemistry* 267 (1992): 15578–84.

Price, Silvia Anderson, and Lorraine McCarty Wilson. *Pathophysiology: Clinical Concepts of Disease Process*. 4th ed. St. Louis, MO: Mosby Year Book, 1992.

Smith, Ed. *Therapeutic Herb Manual*. Williams, OR: Ed Smith, 1999.

Stryer, Lubert. *Biochemistry*. 4th ed. New York: W. H. Freeman & Company, 1995.

Taddei-Ferretti, C., and P. Marotta, eds. *High Dilution Effects on Cells and Integrated Systems*. London: World Scientific, 1998.

Tierra, Michael. *Planetary Herbology*. Twin Lakes, WI: Lotus Press, 1992.

Tortora, Gerard J., and Sandra Reynolds Grabowski. *Principles of Anatomy and Physiology*. 7th ed. New York: HarperCollins, 1993.

Traves, Suzanne L., and Louise E. Donnelly. "Chemokines and Their Receptors as Targets for the Treatment of COPD." *Current Respiratory Medicine Reviews* 1 (2005): 15–32.

Trivieri, Larry, Jr., and John W. Anderson, eds. *Alternative Medicine: The Definitive Guide*. Berkeley, CA: Celestial Arts, 2002.

Uthe, J., and W. Magee. "Phospholipase A2: Action as Affected by Deoxycholate and Divalent Cations." *Canadian Journal of Biochemistry* 49 (1971): 776–84.

West, John B. *Pulmonary Pathophysiology: The Essentials*. 6th ed. Philadelphia: Lippincott, Williams & Wilkins, 2003.

Zuidema, George D., ed. *The Johns Hopkins Atlas of Human Functional Anatomy*. 4th ed. Baltimore: Johns Hopkins University Press, 1997.

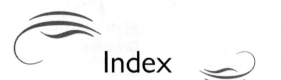

# Index

# BOOKS OF RELATED INTEREST

MEDICAL HERBALISM
*The Science and Practice of Herbal Medicine*
by David Hoffmann, FNIMH, AHG

THE OXYGEN PRESCRIPTION
*The Miracle of Oxidative Therapies*
by Nathaniel Altman

OPTIMAL DIGESTIVE HEALTH: A COMPLETE GUIDE
Edited by Trent W. Nichols, M.D., and Nancy Faass, MSW, MPH

THE ACID–ALKALINE DIET FOR OPTIMUM HEALTH
Restore Your Health by Creating pH Balance in Your Diet
by Christopher Vasey, N.D.

THE WATER PRESCRIPTION
*For Health, Vitality, and Rejuvenation*
by Christopher Vasey, N.D.

THE DETOX MONO DIET
*The Miracle Grape Cure and Other Cleansing Diets*
by Christopher Vasey, N.D.

THE TAO OF DETOX
*The Secrets of Yang-Sheng Dao*
by Daniel Reid

ACUPUNCTURE FOR EVERYONE
*What It Is, Why It Works, and How It Can Help You*
by Dr. Ruth Kidson

Inner Traditions • Bear & Company
P.O. Box 388
Rochester, VT  05767
1-800-246-8648
www.InnerTraditions.com

Or contact your local bookseller